T0252159

PHARMACOTHERAPY
FOR
PSYCHOLOGISTS

PHARMACOTHERAPY FOR PSYCHOLOGISTS

PRESCRIBING AND COLLABORATIVE ROLES

EDITED BY
ROBERT E. McGRATH AND BRET A. MOORE

American Psychological Association • Washington, DC

Published by
American Psychological Association
750 First Street, NE
Washington, DC 20002
www.apa.org

To order
APA Order Department
P.O. Box 92984
Washington, DC 20090-2984
Tel: (800) 374-2721; Direct: (202) 336-5510
Fax: (202) 336-5502; TDD/TTY: (202) 336-6123
Online: www.apa.org/books/
E-mail: order@apa.org

In the U.K., Europe, Africa, and the Middle East, copies may be ordered from
American Psychological Association
3 Henrietta Street
Covent Garden, London
WC2E 8LU England

Typeset in Goudy by Circle Graphics, Inc., Columbia, MD

Printer: Maple-Vail Manufacturing Group, York, PA
Cover Designer: Mercury Publishing Service, Rockville, MD

The opinions and statements published are the responsibility of the authors, and such opinions and statements do not necessarily represent the policies of the American Psychological Association.

Library of Congress Cataloging-in-Publication Data

Pharmacotherapy for psychologists : prescribing and collaborative roles / edited by Robert E. McGrath and Bret A. Moore. — 1st ed.
    p. ; cm.
Includes bibliographical references and index.
ISBN-13: 978-1-4338-0800-5
ISBN-10: 1-4338-0800-5
1. Clinical psychologists—Prescriptive authority. I. McGrath, Robert E., 1956- II. Moore, Bret A. III. American Psychological Association.
    [DNLM: 1. Psychology, Clinical. 2. Drug Prescriptions. 3. Licensure. 4. Mental Disorders—drug therapy. 5. Referral and Consultation. WM 105 P5368 2010]

RC467.97.P53 2010
616.89—dc22
                                        2009052601

British Library Cataloguing-in-Publication Data

A CIP record is available from the British Library.

Printed in the United States of America
First Edition

This is dedicated to my family—
Deb, Megan, and Brian—the three loveliest people I know.
—*Robert E. McGrath*

In memory of Ferrell and Cecelia Abel, Charles Moore, Jack Scobey,
Richard Strait, and Mike Neal.
—*Bret A. Moore*

CONTENTS

Contributors .... *ix*

Foreword: The Challenges of Substantive Change .... *xi*
Patrick H. DeLeon

Acknowledgments .... *xv*

Introduction 3

I. The Roots of the Prescriptive Authority Movement 7

Chapter 1.   Making the Case for Prescriptive Authority 9
              Mark Muse and Robert E. McGrath

Chapter 2.   The Evolution of Training Guidelines
              in Pharmacotherapy for Psychologists 29
              Linda F. Campbell and Ronald Fox

Chapter 3.   The Psychopharmacology Demonstration Project:
              What Did It Teach Us, and Where Are We Now? 49
              Morgan T. Sammons

II. General Practice Issues **69**

Chapter 4.   Nuts and Bolts of Prescriptive Practice 71
               Glenn A. Ally

Chapter 5.   Ethical Considerations in Pharmacotherapy
               for Psychologists 89
               Robert E. McGrath and Beth N. Rom-Rymer

Chapter 6.   Integration of Psychotherapy and Pharmacotherapy
               by Prescribing–Medical Psychologists:
               A Psychobiosocial Model of Care 105
               Elaine S. LeVine and Elaine Orabona Foster

Chapter 7.   Evaluating Drug Research 133
               Robert E. McGrath

III. Settings and Populations **151**

Chapter 8.   In the Private Practice Setting: A Survey
               of the Experiences of Prescribing Psychologists 153
               Elaine S. LeVine and Jack Wiggins

Chapter 9.   Psychologists in Primary Care 173
               Alan R. Gruber

Chapter 10.   Prescribing for School-Aged Patients 189
               Bruce K. McCormick

Chapter 11.   Prescribing in the Public Health Service 207
               Kevin M. McGuinness and Michael R. Tilus

IV. Looking Forward **221**

Chapter 12.   Lessons From the Trenches: Getting Laws Passed 223
               Robert E. McGrath

Chapter 13.   The Future of Prescribing Psychology 233
               Bret A. Moore

Index 241

About the Editors... 255

CONTRIBUTORS

Glenn A. Ally, PhD, MP, ABMP, private practice, Lafayette, LA
Linda F. Campbell, PhD, University of Georgia, Athens
Patrick H. DeLeon, PhD, former president, American Psychological Association
Ronald Fox, PhD, Human Resources Consulting, Chapel Hill, NC
Alan R. Gruber, PhD, NeuroBehavioral Associates, Weymouth, MA
Elaine S. LeVine, PhD, New Mexico State University, Las Cruces
Bruce K. McCormick, PhD, private practice, Shreveport, LA
Bret A. Moore, PsyD, ABPP, Indian Health Service, Poplar, MT
Robert E. McGrath, PhD, Fairleigh Dickinson University, Teaneck, NJ
Kevin M. McGuinness, PhD, MP, ABPP, U.S. Public Health Service, Health Resources and Services Administration, Chaparral, NM
Mark Muse, EdD, ABPP, Muse Psychological Associates, Rockville, MD
Elaine Orabona Foster, PhD, California School of Professional Psychology, Alliant International University, San Francisco, CA
Beth N. Rom-Rymer, PhD, Rom-Rymer & Associates, Chicago, IL
Morgan T. Sammons, PhD, ABPP, California School of Professional Psychology, Alliant International University, San Francisco, CA
Michael R. Tilus, PsyD, U.S. Public Health Service, Fort Totten, ND
Jack Wiggins, PhD, Secretary, Academy of Medical Psychology, Fountain Hills, AZ

FOREWORD: THE CHALLENGES OF SUBSTANTIVE CHANGE

PATRICK H. DELEON

Prescriptive authority, once the exclusive purview of the medical profession in the United States, has expanded rapidly beyond physicians in the past several decades. This expansion has been so dramatic that it is perhaps safe to say that psychosocial, culturally sensitive prescriptive authority represents much of the future for a wide range of nonphysician disciplines. For nonphysician health care professions other than psychology, access to the prescription pad has ensured a rapid—indeed, unprecedented—expansion in their collective scopes of practice. Nurse practitioners, optometrists, podiatrists, and physician assistants are among such professional groups who have seen a dramatic expansion of clinical privileges, largely based on the ability to prescribe drugs. The prescribing of substances designed to produce an effect that counters illness (i.e., allopathy) lies both epistemologically and historically at the center of the practice of medicine. We must remember, however, that a monopoly over control of the prescription pad is a relatively recent—and relatively brief—phenomenon in the history of medicine. It was not until several decades into the 20th century that American physicians were able to restrict this ability to those who held a medical degree. By the 1970s, this monopoly began to be successfully challenged by a number of nonphysician health care professionals. Now, at the end of the first decade of the 21st century, psychology is among the few health care professions, and the only doctoral-level health care profession, that does not possess the universal capability of prescribing drugs.

Thus, prescriptive authority represents a unique opportunity for the profession of psychology to seriously address society's most pressing needs and in so doing, to demonstrate that it is, in fact, a bona fide health care profession, providing high-quality psychopharmacological care from a fundamentally different perspective than those trained in a medical background. It has long been my contention that the practice of clinical psychopharmacology from a psychological perspective will differ substantially from psychopharmacological practice by those trained in the medical model. The psychological model, in brief, is based more on functional than pathological assessments of a patient's condition; views contextual and relational factors to be as important as, if not more important than, neurobiological disturbances in the production of most mental disorders; and does not view psychotropic drugs as standalone curative agents. Time, as well as an increasing number of prescribing psychologists, will determine if this fundamentally different perspective will provide an improvement in available mental health services, but we believe that early indications are positive. From a health policy perspective, then, prescriptive authority for psychologists provides our nation with a viable alternative to traditional medically dominated mental health care—which all of the evidence, over the years, clearly suggests has not been adequate, if for no other reason than access to psychiatric services has not been able to meet the demands for such services. I also believe that prescriptive authority will be a critical catalyst for our next generation of clinicians who are obtaining excellent and meaningful employment opportunities, through an expanded scope of practice that takes advantage of the entirety of an appropriately trained psychologist's clinical training. Simply stated, I believe that obtaining prescriptive authority will significantly improve the quality of care provided to our patients and ensure that psychology is recognized throughout the 21st century health care environment as a respected and necessary discipline.

Psychology's prescriptive-authority quest represents profound and fundamental change. The process of developing appropriate training experiences for our next generation of colleagues to effectively use prescriptive authority will undoubtedly result in many within academia and the American Psychological Association governance taking a close look at the underlying mission of our current university-based training programs. As members of one of the "learned professions," we must ask, Are our training institutions really utilizing society's precious resources to adequately train students for the evolving health care needs of the future, or are these institutions, which are generally supported by tax revenues, merely continuing the status quo by operating within isolated professional silos? Are our scientists and clinical researchers missing out on an exciting opportunity by being less than supportive of the field advancing into this arena? As scientists who represent many of our nation's health care professions seek to advance their collective knowledge in such complex areas as comparative effectiveness research and developing patient-centered clinical protocols, is psychology instead striving to maintain the unfortunate historical separation between "mind and body," primarily due to professional comfort with the status quo?

A dispassionate analysis of the arguments frequently proffered outside of the profession for why psychology should not obtain prescriptive authority provides little support for such objections. In addition, given the persistent problems of access to comprehensive mental health services, does such an analysis lend credence to the argument that our opponents are genuinely thinking about the common good? All of us within psychology should be absolutely clear that we can learn, and many of us have learned, how to effectively utilize psychotropic medications in a cost-effective and culturally sensitive manner. As the authors in this impressive volume have unequivocally documented, there really can be no serious doubt as to the validity of this underlying assertion. We must recall that any perceived encroachment on the scope of practice of physicians by any other health care profession has raised the alarm of a hazard to public safety. Yet this fear has never, under any circumstance, been realized. Accordingly, I would suggest that such arguments are based on a concern for professional authority (i.e., power), prestige, economics, and an underlying fear of the unknown. The research literature on cognitive dissonance is quite relevant to the emotional intensity of medicine's consistent opposition to psychology (and other health professions) in expanding its scope of clinical practice (i.e., "If I had to go to medical school to learn . . . "). Appreciation of the implications and benefits of educated consumers being active partners in determining their own health care protocols would seem far from their minds. It is therefore appropriate to ask, Why shouldn't patients have a real choice in providers and in treatment alternatives?

In the more than three decades for which I have been involved in the public policy arena, I have learned that change is always unsettling for those who perceive themselves as being personally affected, especially if it is substantive in nature. Further, meaningful change always takes much longer than one might have anticipated. I have also learned that once those involved in fostering change focus their efforts on its inherent importance, it evolves over time. There is no question in my mind that psychology has seriously undertaken its quest for obtaining prescriptive authority and that we will succeed. Sometimes, in retrospect, one realizes that by merely waiting for those without vision to retire from the scene, one finds that the next generation simply does not understand why the sought-after modifications have not already been implemented.

ACKNOWLEDGMENTS

Bret A. Moore would like to thank his wife, Lori, for her undying patience and encouragement and his parents, David and Brynda Moore, and brothers, David and Keith Moore, for their support and counsel.

Robert E. McGrath would like to acknowledge the pioneers who made this story possible, particularly Pat DeLeon, Ron Fox, and Jack Wiggins; the participants in the Psychopharmacology Demonstration Project program; and the New Mexico and Louisiana gangs who have watered the seed from one end of this country to the other.

We also would also like to thank Maureen Adams and Beth Hatch of the American Psychological Association who provided guidance and direction throughout the process.

PHARMACOTHERAPY
FOR
PSYCHOLOGISTS

INTRODUCTION

BRET A. MOORE AND ROBERT E. MCGRATH

Pharmacotherapy is perhaps the most quickly evolving area of professional psychology. Within the past few years, psychologists in private practice have begun prescribing psychotropic medications in two states, and a new generation of psychologists is now eligible to prescribe in the military, the U.S. Public Health Service, and the Indian Health Service. More than a dozen states have concluded that consulting on psychotropic medications falls within the scope of practice of psychology, and more than a dozen states have active legislative agendas focused on gaining prescriptive authority for appropriately trained psychologists.

As a result of this progress, psychologists have become increasingly aware of issues surrounding prescriptive authority, including the mechanics of prescriptive practice and the ancillary legal and professional issues associated with functioning as a prescriber. Psychologists lobbying for prescriptive authority have used increasingly sophisticated arguments and strategies to support their efforts. Entities within the American Psychological Association have been considering the implications of psychologists' relationships with the pharmaceutical industry, ethical issues surrounding prescription and collaboration, and training guidelines. Undoubtedly, the movement for prescriptive authority will succeed. The prescriptive authority train has left the station. It is only a matter of where the train stops and how we can create a more comfortable, efficient, and expeditious ride.

WHY PSYCHOLOGISTS SHOULD CARE ABOUT PRESCRIPTIVE AUTHORITY

Proponents of prescriptive authority for psychologists are able to detail a litany of reasons why this evolving area of professional psychology is important to the field. Although other chapters in this volume deal with these issues in more detail, it is reasonable to highlight the most salient here.

First, adding pharmacotherapy to a psychologist's scope of practice provides the psychologist with a greater ability to provide more comprehensive, individually targeted, and effective behavioral health treatment. Psychologists are already trained in counseling and psychotherapy, psychological testing and diagnostics, consultation, consumption and production of research, and supervision. The addition of pharmacological management and increased awareness and understanding of presentations of physical disease creates the consummate behavioral health practitioner. One only needs to look at current training programs in psychiatry to understand that the scope of practice of psychiatry has narrowed and the need for this consummate practitioner is great.

Second, a shift is currently happening within the field of psychology that makes prescriptive authority particularly appropriate. The 50-min therapy session is giving way to targeted 15- to 20-min psychological interventions in the primary care clinic. Understandably, many within the profession are rebelling against this shift. However, others recognize that involvement in a primary care clinic increases access to patients and that secondary and tertiary prevention are effective and can greatly improve the quality of a patient's life. Combining medication management with brief psychological interventions in primary-care settings creates great possibilities for psychologists.

Last, all professions evolve. Psychiatric nursing has evolved into a profession almost completely independent of psychiatry. Licensed counselors are conducting psychological testing. Social workers have moved from conducting social needs assessment and case management to providing direct psychotherapy, with reimbursement rates comparable with those of psychologists. Psychiatrists have moved into more traditional medical settings, providing consultation and liaison services; more and more they are increasing their expertise in neuroimaging, genetics, and nonpharmacological treatments, such as electroconvulsive therapy and psychosurgery. In short, either professional psychology evolves or it risks becoming irrelevant as time passes. Prescriptive authority is the evolution within professional psychology with the greatest potential for markedly changing the way psychologists do business.

RISKS OF PRESCRIPTIVE AUTHORITY

Even the most loyal proponent of prescriptive authority is able to recognize the risks associated with this professional evolution. One of the main arguments by opponents of prescriptive authority is that prescribing psychologists will lose our professional identity and become "junior psychiatrists." Although the term is rather demeaning, there is some validity to the concern about whether prescribing psychologists will neglect psychosocial interventions for pharmacological ones. One way to mitigate this possibility is to ensure that all doctoral students in clinical psychology and related disciplines receive exposure to psychopharmacology, as recommended by Smyer et al. (1993). This way, all psychologists have the basic foundation that will allow them to consult with prescribing health care providers while retaining their traditional identities as providers of psychological treatments. A student should not be forced to "join a camp" with regard to prescriptive authority— that is, either undergoing all necessary training to become certified to prescribe or neglecting the study of pharmacology altogether. Rather, doctoral students in psychology should be given the knowledge necessary to choose whether to continue with training in psychopharmacology in order to add medication management or consultation to their toolbox or whether to develop and hone nonpharmacological interventions at the postdoctoral level. Forcing any one identity on someone will likely backfire, particularly within a profession that is itself undergoing significant identity change.

To ignore the less than altruistic reasons why some psychologists are interested in obtaining prescriptive authority is to risk the sincerity and credibility of the movement. Without question, proponents of prescriptive authority are concerned about the lack of timely and appropriate psychiatric services available to citizens. They understand the common sense behind patients having the choice to see one provider for both psychological and pharmacological interventions. They wholeheartedly believe that the power to prescribe is also the power to not prescribe or to unprescribe. These are the mainstay beliefs behind the prescriptive authority movement. However, it is counterproductive to dismiss entirely claims by opponents that the prescriptive authority movement is motivated by financial factors. The truth is that prescriptive authority will likely bring greater financial rewards to psychologists who prescribe. We can even expect that for a segment of psychologists who pursue prescriptive authority, increased compensation is a primary motivator. However, the financial incentive for psychologists to pursue prescriptive authority is no different from the financial incentive for researchers to pursue research funding, or for students to become licensed psychologists in the first place. Doing well for society and doing well for oneself are not mutually exclusive. Pretending that they are contradicts common sense and human nature and dampens the credibility of prescriptive authority proponents by conveying a false hyperbenevolence, which legislators most surely can detect. Most important, to pursue prescriptive authority at least in part for financial gain does not undermine its pursuit for altruistic reasons as well.

THE CURRENT VOLUME

This volume provides a snapshot of the professional issues surrounding prescriptive authority, medical collaboration, and practical issues associated with prescribing. It will be useful to those involved in legislative efforts, psychologists who are considering completing the training required to become a medical or prescribing psychologist, and those currently prescribing. It will also be a resource for those who do not decide to pursue prescriptive authority but are interested in becoming better collaborators around medication issues with those who do prescribe.

The book comprises four parts. Part I covers the rationale for prescriptive authority (Chapter 1) and key issues in the history of the prescriptive authority movement, including the most recent training guidelines used today (Chapter 2) and the Department of Defense Psychopharmacology Demonstration Project (Chapter 3). More general histories of the prescriptive authority movement are already available elsewhere (see Fox, 2003; McGrath, in press). Part II covers general practice issues, including the challenges of day-to-day pharmacotherapy practice (Chapter 4), ethical considerations of pharmacotherapy (Chapter 5), the integration of psychotherapy and pharmacotherapy (Chapter 6), and the evaluation of drug research (Chapter 7). Part III describes issues related to prescribing in specific settings and with specific populations, including private practice (Chapter 8), primary care clinics (Chapter 9), schools (Chapter 10), and public health agencies (Chapter 11). Finally, Part IV provides ideas for getting prescriptive authority laws passed (Chapter 12) and the future of prescribing psychology (Chapter 13).

REFERENCES

Fox, R. E. (2003). Early efforts by psychologists to obtain prescriptive authority. In M. T. Sammons, R. U. Paige, & R. F. Levant (Eds.), *Prescriptive authority for psychologists: A history and guide* (pp. 33–45). Washington, DC: American Psychological Association. doi:10.1037/10484-002

McGrath, R. E. (in press). Prescriptive authority for psychologists. *Annual Review of Clinical Psychology*.

Smyer, M. A., Balster, R. L., Egli, D., Johnson, D. L., Kilbey, M. M., Leith, N. J., & Puente, A. E. (1993). Summary of the report of the ad hoc task force on psychopharmacology of the American Psychological Association. *Professional Psychology, Research and Practice, 24,* 394–403. doi:10.1037/0735-7028.24.4.394

I

THE ROOTS OF THE PRESCRIPTIVE AUTHORITY MOVEMENT

1

MAKING THE CASE FOR PRESCRIPTIVE AUTHORITY

MARK MUSE AND ROBERT E. McGRATH

This chapter summarizes the arguments in favor of, and counters the arguments against, awarding psychologists prescriptive authority. Regardless of whether one supports psychologists' efforts to become prescribers, is uncertain or neutral on the topic, or opposes those efforts, it is important to understand the reasons why many psychologists have become strong advocates for the cause. It is our hope that this chapter will help supporters crystallize their thinking on the topic, those with mixed feelings to see the value of the prescriptive authority movement, and opponents to reconsider their position.

This chapter begins with a summary of the arguments for prescriptive authority for psychologists, followed by a response to the arguments against. In brief, the former set of arguments reduces to the issue of access, whereas the latter arguments have to do with safety. If the case can be made that prescriptive authority for psychologists improves access to appropriate care without compromising safety, then from a logical perspective the correct position on this controversy is the following: Psychologists should be allowed to prescribe.

THE CASE FOR PRESCRIPTIVE AUTHORITY

Kessler et al. (2005) concluded that although the prevalence and severity of mental disorders in the adult population ages 18 to 54 was stable at about 30% between 1990 and 2003, and although the rate of treatment for those disorders increased by about 60%, more than two thirds of individuals who suffered with a mental disorder still reported they received no treatment. Census figures suggest this translates into approximately 15 million adults who could benefit from specialized mental health services. Furthermore, among those who received treatment, the most common treatment setting was a general medical practice without concomitant specialty services (Wang et al., 2006). Prospective studies that evaluate the prevalence of mental disorders among children ages 9 to 16 similarly tend to suggest rates of 36% to 39% (Jaffee et al., 2005), and it is reasonable to hypothesize that treatment patterns are similar. Clearly, there is a need for expanded specialty mental health care. Yet the availability of psychiatric care is shrinking. Rao (2003) found a 36.5% decline in the number of psychiatric residents over the period 1992 to 2000. Another sign that psychiatry was not attracting sufficient numbers was Rao's finding that during the same period the percentage of psychiatric residents who were graduates of foreign versus U.S. medical schools increased from 27.3% to 41.6%.

The lack of psychiatrists affects potential consumers of mental health services primarily in two ways. First, psychopharmacotherapy is usually delivered in primary care settings by practitioners without specialty training in psychiatric diagnosis and psychotropic medications (Beardsley, Gardocki, Larson, & Hildalgo, 1988; Pincus et al., 1998). A recent survey found that both urban and rural psychologists identified medication management to be the most common unmet need among individuals with mental disorders (Campbell, Kearns, & Patchin, 2006). Second, shortages in appropriate specialty care are not distributed equally across the general population. The economically disadvantaged, members of ethnic and cultural minorities, and individuals living in rural settings particularly find appropriate care difficult to access as a result of multiple factors, such as lack of insurance and geographic isolation.

Access for the Underserved

At the core of the altruistic argument for prescriptive authority of psychologists (RxP) is the effort to reach the underserved with services that are, in many cases, unattainable for them at present. Since the inception of the movement, proponents of prescriptive authority for psychologists have considered meeting the needs of underserved populations as a core rationale (DeLeon, Fox, & Graham, 1991). This would seem to be particularly evident in the case of Hawaii, where a bill was submitted to enable prescriptive authority specifically for isolated indigenous groups treated in a network of 13 federally funded health clinics, offering primary care to the poor and underinsured (Munsey, 2006). The Indian Health Service has also been trying to employ psychologists with prescriptive authority to serve Native Americans living on reservations, who often have no psychiatric services available to them (McGrath, 2008).

Psychiatrists have not done a good job of meeting the needs of the underserved if the number of rural counties without any psychiatrist in residence is used as a measure. For example, recent testimony to the California Senate indicated that 11 of 58 counties in the state are without psychiatrists and 17 more are served by five or fewer psychiatrists. Furthermore, agencies meeting the needs of underserved populations are competing over those psychiatrists who are willing to work in such agencies, as illustrated by a recent article indicating that many psychiatrists have abandoned urban clinics and state hospitals that serve primarily low-income populations for more lucrative contracts with California prisons (Romney, 2007). Still, it might be argued that psychologists with prescriptive authority will tend to serve urban and affluent populations and may no better meet the needs of the underserved than have psychiatrists traditionally.

Although there is credence to the argument that some psychologists with prescriptive authority may continue to serve in settings where lack of access to appropriate care has never been an issue, the differences in the number and distribution of psychologists and psychiatrists will contribute to filling service gaps elsewhere. Whereas there are 14.6 psychiatrists per 100,000 residents in U.S. urban areas and only 3.9 per 100,000 in rural areas, there are 20 psychologists per 100,000 in urban areas and 15 per 100,000 in rural areas (Hartley, Bird, & Dempsey, 1999). Awarding prescriptive authority to psychologists could double the availability of specialty care with psychotropic medications in urban settings, but it potentially increases availability in rural areas sixfold. The recent prescriptive authority bill submitted in Tennessee, which calls for supervised clinical training to be completed in a federally qualified health center, provides an example of the innovative approaches psychologists are pursuing to improve access to care.

Nonetheless, now that psychologists are being awarded prescriptive authority, it is important to demonstrate that they are in fact providing services to the underserved, that access to care is not a whimsical speculation or an ephemeral ploy to gain professional advantage. To this purpose, we surveyed currently prescribing civilian psychologists in those jurisdictions where prescriptive authority has been attained. We queried 18 prescribing or conditionally prescribing psychologists licensed in New Mexico and 45 medical psychologists licensed in Louisiana. Of the 63 individuals sent the survey, 26 responded—10 from New Mexico (56% return rate) and 16 from Louisiana (36% return rate).

On average, civilian psychologists with prescriptive authority estimated that over half of the clients they serve are disadvantaged in one way or another, although the distribution varies across the two states (see Table 1.1). Economically disadvantaged persons represent the single largest category regardless of jurisdiction. It is not surprising that geographic isolation and linguistic barriers are more prevalent in New Mexico, a state characterized by remote communities including Indian reservations and a sizable Spanish-speaking population.

TABLE 1.1
Average Responses to Survey

Question	New Mexico Overall *M* (%)	Louisiana Overall *M* (%)	Total Combined *M* (%)
1. Please estimate the overall percentage of your clientele that is "disadvantaged"	66	47	55
Economically (e.g., under poverty level)	59	36	46
Socially (e.g., educational and/or work opportunities)	24	20	25
Geographically (e.g., rural isolation or urban isolation)	32	10	20
Legally (e.g., incarcerated, irregular immigration)	4	4	4
Linguistically (e.g., non-English speaking)	8	2	5
2. Please estimate the overall percentage increase in disadvantaged population since obtaining prescriptive authority.	26	18	22
3. Do you have any plans to increase your dedication with the underserved and/or underprivileged (e.g., set up a clinic or office for such purposes, offer more pro bono, or expand current availability for such referrals)?	Yes: 75	Yes: 33	Yes: 50
4. How important was serving the underprivileged in your motivation to undergo RxP training and licensing?			
No. 1 priority	40	14	27
Secondary consideration	60	57	55
Not considered	0	29	18

Respondents were also asked to estimate the increase, since acquiring prescriptive authority, in the percentage of patients seen who demonstrate some form of disadvantage (see Table 1.1). The mean estimate is slightly higher for New Mexico than for Louisiana. Several Louisianan prescribing psychologists, however, indicated they initially were finding it difficult to gain entry to community mental health centers and were denied reimbursement under Medicaid. The latter restriction was lifted in May 2008. Despite such obstacles, psychologists reported they have seen the number of disadvantage patients they see increase by one fifth since obtaining prescriptive authority. The report of prescribing psychologists would indicate they are either being sought out by, or are actively seeking out, disadvantaged patients that they would not otherwise have seen were they not practicing pharmacotherapy.

A more marked difference was evident between jurisdictions on whether prescribing psychologists plan to increase services to the disadvantaged further (see Table 1.1). Though psychologists in New Mexico on average reported a larger relative increase in the number of disadvantaged individuals they serve since receiving prescriptive authority in 2002, they also were far more likely to report they plan to increase service to the disadvantaged more. Despite the differences, half of all currently practicing psychologists with prescriptive authority reported that they expect to increase the percentage of disadvantaged patients whom they serve.

Serving the underprivileged was a motivator for undergoing psychopharmacology training in 82% of all currently licensed prescribing psychologists who responded to the survey. In the state of New Mexico, 100% of those psychologists who are currently prescribing were motivated to some degree to undergo psychopharmacology training to better serve the disadvantaged. More than one in three New Mexican respondents indicated that providing greater access to the underserved was the principal reason for undergoing psychopharmacology training.

Respondents were also given the opportunity to add comments to the form about the reasons they chose to pursue prescriptive authority, and those comments highlighted the differences seen between the two jurisdictions in regard to access to treatment. While New Mexico psychologists tended to emphasize extending pharmacotherapy to less fortunate segments of the population, Louisiana psychologists more frequently commented on providing greater access for the population as a whole. The issue of quality of care is addressed next.

Improving Quality of Care

Providing all Americans greater access to quality integrated mental health services—services in which treatment plans are based on a broad spectrum of empirically based biological, social, and psychological options—is considered by most of its supporters to be the primary driving force behind the movement for prescriptive authority for psychologists. The prescriptive authority movement is based on the proposition that quality of care can be improved by increasing access overall and by providing a fully integrated mental health approach to those patients seen by prescribing psychologists. Psychologists are in a unique position to offer an integrated approach to care given their combined training in assessment and evaluation, diagnosis, psychosocial interventions, and now prescriptive authority.

That most Americans who meet criteria for a mental disorder, and for that matter most citizens of developed nations in need of treatment for emotional symptoms (Muse, 2007), do not receive such integrated care is evidenced in the statistics showing that the majority of mental health needs are dealt with in the primary care consulting room and that most psychopharmaceuticals are prescribed by primary care physicians (Beardsley et al., 1988; Pincus et al., 1998).

Primary care providers are subject to three particularly important limitations as providers of mental health care. First, a basic premise in medicine is that a proper diagnosis is essential to effective intervention. Research consistently demonstrates that primary care physicians underdiagnose the frequency of mental and behavioral disorders in the populations they serve (e.g., Richardson, Keller, Selby-Harrington, & Parrish, 1996; Williams-Russo, 1996). It is also likely that without extensive training in issues that surround psychiatric diagnosis they rely heavily on the self-report of the patient to decide on an appropriate course of treatment without considering alternative or comorbid conditions.

Second, given the brevity of office visits with physicians (Mechanic, McAlpine, & Rosenthal, 2001), it is questionable whether primary care physicians will ever be in a position to offer adequate diagnostic services for individuals with mental disorders. Finally, physicians without extensive training in and experience with psychosocial interventions tend to rely on medications as their only formal intervention for mental disorders (Wang et al., 2006). Indeed, evidence suggests even psychiatrists have reduced and continue to reduce further their use of psychosocial interventions (Mojtabai & Olfson, 2008).

The increased availability of integrative care that results from awarding psychologists prescriptive authority has a number of benefits.[1] These benefits include allowing the psychologist an enhanced role as a collaborator with the

---

[1]One should not be misled by the term *prescriptive authority* when psychologists really seek *medication management*, something that is not synonymous with prescribing because in many cases where medication use is not supported by evidence the prescribing psychologist would instead opt to prescribe a nonpharmacological treatment.

patient on the coordination of care across specialist medical providers, fewer visits to multiple professionals and therefore greater efficiency, and more consistent messages to patients about the role of psychotherapy in their treatment. Legislators and the general public are increasingly concerned that the medical establishment has become overly reliant on medication, and the case can be made that psychologists extensively trained in all modalities of treatment are less likely to rely on medication (Wiggins & Cummings, 1998). Growing the number of providers could result in cost savings, as research suggests that nonphysician prescribers can reduce costs by 15% (Speer & Bess, 2003). Finally, it increases the potential for the integration of pharmacotherapy and psychotherapy as research increasingly identifies circumstances in which psychotherapy or combined treatment are superior to pharmacotherapy alone (e.g., Brown et al., 2008; Fabiano et al., 2007; Sammons & Schmidt, 2003; Walkup et al., 2008).

Increased access and freedom of choice are the core issues involved in quality of care. Patients, whether disadvantaged or not, are best served by full-spectrum mental health treatment that addresses the entire biopsychosocial parameters of the patient's condition. Such choice is not generally available, nor is it likely to be without prescriptive authority for qualified providers from diverse professional backgrounds. To insist that only physicians can write prescriptions for psychoactive medications is to support the suboptimal standard of care that defines current practice.

COUNTERING THE CASE AGAINST PRESCRIPTIVE AUTHORITY

Opponents of prescriptive authority for psychologists often raise three variants of the safety argument in testimony to and discussions with legislators (American Psychiatric Association Division of Government Relations, 2003):

1. Psychologists who want to prescribe should go to medical school.
2. The Department of Defense's Psychopharmacology Demonstration Project (PDP), which is the only program training psychologists to prescribe that has been evaluated, was a failure.
3. Psychologists who do not graduate from medical school would not be safe prescribers.

These arguments are addressed one at a time in the following subsections.

Medical School Argument

The argument that psychologists should attend medical school if they want to prescribe can be addressed in several ways. First, it subverts the principal justification for seeking prescriptive authority for psychologists, which is to increase substantially the number of appropriately trained prescribers of psychotropic medications to fill gaps in access to care. If medical schools were to open up ample additional training slots, some psychologists might well opt for that avenue of training, but such an increase in the availability of training is unlikely to occur. Furthermore, it is an inefficient route because much of medical school training (and nursing training, in the case of the psychiatric nurse practitioner) is irrelevant or only tenuously related to the practice of psychopharmacology. To cite just one example, psychiatrists rarely engage in such core medical activities as the physical exam (Krummel & Kathol, 1987; Patterson, 1978).

The real error in this argument, however, is the presumption that only medical schools can train adequate prescribers. Physicians have argued this point, and lost, against advanced practice nurses, optometrists, podiatrists, and clinical pharmacists. There is nothing magical about medical school. The same curriculum can be taught and learned outside of medical faculties. In fact, this *must* be the case if we are to meet the expanding health needs of the general population (McGrath & Muse, 2010).

Research provides no evidence that the competence of physicians as prescribers is superior to that of nonphysician prescribers. Research has demonstrated that nurse practitioners and other nonphysician prescribers offer more educational and counseling services than physicians (e.g., Hooker & McCaig, 2001) and that outcomes are equivalent to those for physicians (Lenz, Mundinger, Kane, Hopkins, & Lin, 2004; Mundinger et al., 2000; U.S. Congress, Office of Technology Assessment, 1986). In addition, patient acceptance of nonphysician-prescribing providers has generally been high (Cooper, 2001).

If a medical degree is not necessary to achieve competence as a prescriber, as the research suggests, if it is arguably an inefficient path for increasing access to safe and effective care, then the real question becomes, Are psychologists adequately trained to prescribe? The answer to this question is found in comparing psychopharmacologically trained psychologists with members of other professions who are currently authorized to prescribe and are, ipso facto, considered to be adequately trained. To this end, we conducted a study (Muse & McGrath, 2010) to highlight the similarities and differences among prescribing mental health professionals' academic preparation. Table 1.2 compares the training of psychologists who are preparing to prescribe with that of other prescribing professions, with special attention paid to those professions most likely to prescribe psychotropics.

Table 1.2 demonstrates that psychologists are among the most highly educated of all health care providers with prescriptive authority. After completing what is usually at least 5 years of graduate training in preparation for the doctor-

TABLE 1.2
Comparison of Training Models

Profession	Minimum years post-baccalaureate	Graduate contact hours M (SD)						
		Biochemistry–Neuroscience	Pharmacology	Clinical practicum	Research statistics	Behavioral assessment–diagnosis & psychometrics	Psychosocial interventions–psychotherapy	Other mental health–psychology course work
Nursing[a]	2.5	48 (7)	56 (7)	146 (33)	99 (41)	30 (23)	32 (29)	128 (77)
Medicine[b]	4	216 (20)	59 (28)	855 (101)	33 (20)	18 (25)	9 (20)	15 (21)
Psychology[c]	6.5	161 (43)	288 (63)	680 (83)	225 (64)	267 (61)	255 (161)	351 (152)

Note. Values were computed equating one academic credit with 15 contact hours.
[a]Based on nurse practitioner master's degree programs at the Medical University of North Carolina, St. Joseph's College, University of Virginia, Vanderbilt University, and Yale University.
[b]Based on medical doctor or doctor of osteopathy programs without residency at the Mayo College of Medicine, Yale University, Tufts University, Stanford University, and A.T. Still University.
[c]Based on doctor of medicine, doctor of education, or doctor of psychology programs plus the postdoctoral master of science program at Alliant University, Fairleigh Dickinson University, the Massachusetts School of Professional Psychology, New Mexico State University, and NOVA Southeastern University.

ate, including coursework, comprehensive exams, dissertation and internship, prescribing psychologists continue their studies for another 2 to 3 years in clinical psychopharmacology, and they must pass a rigorous national comprehensive examination called the Psychopharmacology Examination for Psychologists. New Mexico requires substantially more practicum hours than the number specified in the American Psychological Association's (2008) model curriculum for prescriptive authority, extending the training several years before the psychologist is eligible to prescribe independently. Medical psychologists undergo more training directly relevant to prescribing psychotropics than any other health care professional in Table 1.2, including physicians who hold an MD or DO degree, before they are eligible to prescribe.

In addition to making manifest the greater training that medical psychologists receive in pharmacology than do their nursing and physician colleagues, Table 1.2 presents, in the last four columns, a uniquely psychological perspective on what competencies are relevant to becoming a competent prescriber. The marked difference in the number of hours devoted to research methodology raises the question of whether physicians are optimally qualified to evaluate the research base for the efficacy of the products that they prescribe, or to critically evaluate arguments from drug representatives about the efficacy and safety of the drugs that they prescribe (Healy, 2004). Similarly, psychologists' unique training in behavioral health assessment and measurement sets them apart from any of the other paths toward prescribing. The concern over misdiagnosis and overdiagnosis in mental health (e.g., Bisserbe, Weiller, Boyer, Lépine, & Lecrubier, 1996; Fleet et al., 1996; Leon et al., 1995), leading at times to overmedicating (Hohmann, 1989; Linden et al., 1999; van der Waals, Mohrs, & Foet, 1993), by itself raises concerns about prescribing without a firm background in psychological assessment as a tool for challenging or validating cursory clinical impressions about a patient.

The final two columns of the table present a comparison of the amount of education and training that the professions most likely to prescribe psychotropics receive in the area of alternative interventions to medications, as well as in foundation areas that provide a broad understanding of mental health issues. It goes without saying that medication is only one modality of intervention in the treatment of mental, emotional, and behavioral disorders, and that the ability to accurately diagnose and offer the most appropriate intervention is the crux of being a well-rounded mental health professional. The more extensive training psychologists receive in psychological foundations, mental health theory, and psychosocial management of behavioral concerns increases the likelihood that medication will be viewed in a larger context, rather than as the treatment of choice in all circumstances. In contrast to the primary care physician, who must remain current in a wide array of domains, the psychologist is in a better position to remain current in the spectrum of treatment options available for mental disorders, a necessary condition for the implementation of evidence-based behavioral medicine.

One does not have to go to medical school to be a well-informed, safe, and effective prescriber. In fact, the medical school model has limitations in terms of cost and efficiency. When compared with typical standards of what is considered adequate training for prescriptive authority, the postdoctoral-training psychologists receive is consistent with that of other disciplines and, indeed, is superior in many of the academic content areas that should comprise part of the education of a well-informed mental health prescriber. When opponents argue that training for prescriptive authority among psychologists is inadequate (e.g., Heiby, 2010), they are ignoring the broad array of content domains relevant to optimal practice.

PDP Argument

The PDP is described in some detail in Chapter 3 of this volume. Opponents of prescriptive authority for psychologists have often argued before state legislatures that the PDP represents the only circumstances under which prescriptive authority for psychologists has been evaluated, and the program proved to be a failure. As evidence for this conclusion they are inclined to cite the U. S. General Accounting Office's (GAO; 1997, 1999) assessment of the PDP. In fact, the documents substantiate the high level of knowledge-based expertise and clinical skills of the prescribing psychologists: the safety record of the graduates was undisputed. The criticisms of the program, as outlined by the GAO, were unrelated to safety or efficacy issues. The GAO found two shortcomings of the program, both of which were unique that the PDP: (a) the cost of training the participating psychologists was too high; and (b) there was little effect on military readiness because there were so few participants and because psychotropic medications generally do not represent the treatment of choice in wartime.

The first criticism can be addressed in several ways. It should be noted that the costs referenced encompassed start-up and program evaluation. Second, part of the cost reflected a curriculum that initially mirrored several years of medical school. We have already raised the argument that this approach to training is excessive and cost inefficient. In fact, the curriculum of the PDP was drastically reduced during the life span of the program (Sammons & Brown, 1997). Finally, since termination of PDP all three branches of the military offering health care services (Air Force, Army, and Navy) have developed regulations that formally permit awarding prescribing privileges to psychologists who have received, and paid for out of pocket, psychopharmacological training in civilian educational institutions.

In response to the second criticism, it should be noted that the PDP was established during peacetime. Since then, prescribing psychologists—including several PDP graduates—have served in both Iraq and Afghanistan (e.g., Hopewell, 2008; Moore, 2008; Younger, 2007a, 2007b). Dr. Alan Hopewell was awarded the Bronze Star for his role as a frontline provider in the Iraq conflict ("Prescribing Psychologist in Iraq Awarded Bronze Star Medal," 2008).

The PDP program has been called "one of the most intensively studied and widely scrutinized experiments in the training of non-physicians for prescriptive authority" (Newman, Phelps, Sammons, Dunivin, & Cullen, 2000, p. 598), having undergone four full-scale evaluations by the time it was terminated. A preliminary evaluation was conducted at the behest of the Assistant Secretary of Defense for Health Affairs (Vector Research, 1996). Unlike the GAO, Vector Research excluded one-time start-up costs and found that training psychologists to prescribe would be substantially cheaper on a yearly basis than training physicians. A fourth and final evaluation, and the most extensive evaluation of the set, was that of the American College of Neuropsychopharmacology (ACNP; 1991, 1998). Despite preliminary concerns about the feasibility of training psychologists to prescribe without physician oversight, the final report (ACNP, 1998) ultimately concluded that

> PDP graduates have performed and are performing safely and effectively as prescribing psychologists. . . . it seems clear to the Evaluation Panel that a 2-year program—one year didactic, one year clinical practicum that includes at least a 6-month inpatient rotation—can transform licensed clinical psychologists into prescribing psychologists who can function effectively and safely in the military setting to expand the delivery of mental health treatment to a variety of patients and clients in a cost effective way. As such, we are in agreement that the Psychopharmacology Demonstration Project is a job well done. (p. 6)

Safety Argument

Perhaps the most direct argument used against prescriptive authority for psychologists suggests that psychologists would be unsafe prescribers. One example of this strategy to discredit is recounted by Tim Duke, PsyD (and now MD), one of the PDP graduates:

> When I testified in front of the Missouri state legislature in 1999, one of the arguments that a practicing psychiatrist presented to the subcommittee was that psychologists would not know how to handle or identify such horrible diseases as Steven-Johnson's syndrome. . . . I suggested to the committee that any individual at any educational level who saw a person walking around with blisters all over their body would come to the conclusion that the person was sick and needed care and, furthermore, psychiatry would not be taking care of this person. (T. Duke, personal communication, April 22, 2008)

The evidence for the safety of nonphysician prescribers in general was reviewed earlier. More immediately relevant is informal data available from the 15 years of prescribing in the military, by providers in all three branches of military who have written thousands of prescriptions in both times of peace and time of war and from the thousands of prescriptions that have been written by psychologists in Louisiana and New Mexico since the institution of prescriptive authority in those jurisdictions. To date, there is no evidence that any major adverse event has resulted from a prescription written by a prescribing psychologist. To our knowledge—and as of this writing—no complaint has ever been filed concerning a prescribing psychologist with either a state licensing board or the company that provides malpractice insurance specifically for prescribers, the American Psychological Association Insurance Trust. Prescribing psychologists have safely prescribed for children, adolescents, adults, and geriatric patients; in children's hospitals, general hospitals, rehabilitation facilities, psychiatric hospitals, private practices, and outpatient clinics; acting in the capacity of provider, department head, clinical supervisors, and preceptors to family medicine residents; within state, federal, and private service; and overseas in Iraq, Afghanistan, Kuwait, and Germany, as well as at sea; for 15 years within the Department of Defense, 4 years in the state of Louisiana, and 5 years in New Mexico. The argument that RxP psychologists pose a threat to safety is simply not defensible.

COUNTERING PSYCHOLOGISTS' CONCERNS

One group critical to prescriptive authority in particular merits special consideration, that being psychologists opposed to the movement. Many psychologists had initial doubts about pursuing prescriptive authority (Massoth, McGrath, Bianchi, & Singer, 1990), but most have been persuaded with time of the movement's value by the arguments in favor of prescriptive authority for psychologists (Ax, Forbes, & Thompson, 1997; Sammons, Gorny, Zinner, & Allen, 2000; Walters, 2001) and support has continued to increase in more recent surveys (Baird, 2007; Fagan et al., 2004). It is not surprising that younger psychologists are somewhat more in favor of prescriptive authority (St-Pierre & Melnyk, 2004), arguing for an even greater support base for the future.

The arguments against prescriptive authority by pensive, cautious psychologists have generally revolved around the fear that such authority would compromise the identity and integrity of the profession by following in the footsteps of psychiatry (e.g., Adams & Bieliauskas, 1994), where psychosocial factors have been relegated to a mere footnote alongside the predominantly biological explanation of emotional disturbance (Mojtabai & Olfson, 2008).

As discussion has ensued on this issue, though, several resiliency factors have been identified that should reaffirm the discipline's psychosocial foundations. Among these are the lower reliance in comparison to psychiatry on foreign graduates who may be uncomfortable with psychosocial treatments that are based largely on cultural and linguistic understanding; and the relegation of psychopharmacology to a postdoctoral training experience only pursued by some psychologists, ensuring that those who pursue further postdoctoral training in pharmacotherapy do so by building on a firm social scientist base. Perhaps one of the most important arguments to assuage the fear that psychology's identity might become compromised in the face of the addition of prescriptive authority is psychology's status as a science, a status that is much broader than psychology as a profession or even psychology as a discipline. The scientist–practitioner is trained to a certain level of skepticism. To the extent that pharmacologic treatment of mental and emotional conditions proves its place in the larger context of therapeutic management of such disorders, there is no need to take an ideological stance or theoretical position for or against it. To the extent that psychosocial interventions are demonstrated to be a useful alternative or adjunct to medications, psychologists are more likely to retain loyalty to those interventions. Such demonstrations will also ensure the continued professional success of psychologists who choose not to pursue prescriptive authority as they, instead, continue to pursue excellence as therapists.

With time, most in the psychological community have come to understand that psychologists who prescribe are not "pill happy" (Wiggins & Cummings, 1998; Wiggins & Wedding, 2004). Some former opponents have recognized that not all psychologists will need to pursue prescriptive authority, and personal disinterest in becoming a prescriber need not imply opposition to those psychologists who are interested. Early concerns about the impact of prescriptive authority on malpractice rates have also been mitigated by the Insurance Trust's announcement that prescribing psychologists will be treated as a separate risk pool.

CONCLUSION

Prescriptive authority for psychologists improves access to optimal care without compromising safety. The demand for adequate mental health care far exceeds its current availability, and psychologists trained to prescribe medication offer a cost-efficient, timely, safe, and effective means for addressing shortages of care. Prescribing psychologists are already making a difference in those jurisdictions where prescriptive authority is available. Prescriptive authority for psychologists will mean improved access to optimal care for all mental health consumers.

REFERENCES

Adams, K. M., & Bieliauskas, L. A. (1994). On perhaps becoming what you had previously despised: Psychologists as prescribers of medication. *Journal of Clinical Psychology in Medical Settings, 1,* 189–197. doi:10.1007/BF01989620

American College of Neuropsychopharmacology. (1991). Prescribing privileges for non-physicians in the military: Accepted as a consensus statement by the ACNP Council, March 22, 1991. *Neuropsychopharmacology, 4,* 290–291.

American College of Neuropsychopharmacology. (1998). *DoD prescribing psychologists: External analysis, monitoring, and evaluation of the program and its participants.* Nashville, TN: Author.

American Psychiatric Association Division of Government Relations. (2003). *Scope of practice: Psychologist prescribing legislation.* Arlington, VA: American Psychiatric Association. Retrieved from http://www.oklahomapsychiatry.org/APA position paper.pdf

American Psychological Association. (2008). *Recommended postdoctoral education and training program in psychopharmacology for prescriptive authority.* Washington, DC: Author.

Ax, R. K., Forbes, M. R., & Thompson, D. D. (1997). Prescription privileges for psychologists: A survey of predoctoral interns and directors of training. *Professional Psychology, Research and Practice, 28,* 509–514. doi:10.1037/0735-7028.28.6.509

Baird, K. A. (2007). A survey of clinical psychologists in Illinois regarding prescription privileges. *Professional Psychology, Research and Practice, 38,* 196–202. doi:10.1037/0735-7028.38.2.196

Beardsley, R.-S., Gardocki, G. J., Larson, D. B., & Hildalgo, J. (1988). Prescribing of psychotropic medication by primary care physicians and psychiatrists. *Archives of General Psychiatry, 45,* 1117–1119.

Bisserbe, J.-C., Weiller, E., Boyer, P., Lépine, J.-P., & Lecrubier, Y. (1996). Social phobia in primary care: Level of recognition and drug use. *International Clinical Psychopharmacology, 11*(Suppl. 3), 25–28. doi:10.1097/00004850-199606003-00005

Brown, R. T., Antonuccio, D. O., DuPaul, G. J., Fristad, M. E., King, C. E., Leslie, L. K., . . . Vitiello, B. (2008). *Childhood mental health disorders: Evidence base and contextual factors for psychosocial, psychopharmacological, and combined interventions.* Washington, DC: American Psychological Association. doi:10.1037/11638-000

Campbell, C. D., Kearns, L. A., & Patchin, S. (2006). Psychological needs and resources as perceived by rural and urban psychologists. *Professional Psychology, Research and Practice, 37,* 45–50. doi:10.1037/0735-7028.37.1.45

Cooper, R. A. (2001). Health care workforce for the twenty-first century: The impact of nonphysician clinicians. *Annual Review of Medicine, 52,* 51–61. doi:10.1146/annurev.med.52.1.51

DeLeon, P. H., Fox, R. E., & Graham, S. R. (1991). Prescription privileges: Psychology's next frontier? *American Psychologist, 46,* 384–393. doi:10.1037/0003-066X.46.4.384

Fabiano, G. A., Pelham, W. E., Jr., Gnagy, E. M., Burrows-MacLean, L., Coles, E. K., Chacko, A., . . . Robb, J. A. (2007). The single and combined effects of multiple intensities of behavior modification and methylphenidate for children with attention deficit hyperactivity disorder in a classroom setting. *School Psychology Review, 36,* 195–216.

Fagan, T. J., Ax, R. K., Resnick, R. J., Liss, M., Johnson, R. T., & Forbes, M. R. (2004). Attitudes among interns and directors of training: Who wants to prescribe, who doesn't, and why. *Professional Psychology, Research and Practice, 35,* 345–356. doi:10.1037/0735-7028.35.4.345

Fleet, R. P., Dupuis, G., Marchand, A., Burelle, D., Arsenault, A., & Beitman, B. D. (1996). Panic disorder in emergency department chest pain patients: Prevalence, comorbidity, suicidal ideation, and physician recognition. *The American Journal of Medicine, 101,* 371–380. doi:10.1016/S0002-9343(96)00224-0

Hartley, D., Bird, D., & Dempsey, P. (1999). Rural mental health and substance abuse. In T. C. Ricketts (Ed.), *Rural health in the United States* (pp. 159–178). New York, NY: Oxford University Press.

Healy, D. (2004). *Let them eat Prozac: The unhealthy relationship between the pharmaceutical industry and depression.* New York, NY: New York University Press.

Heiby, E. M. (2010). Concerns about substandard training for prescription privileges for psychologists. *Journal of Clinical Psychology, 66,* 104–111.

Hohmann, A. A. (1989). Gender bias in psychotropic drug prescribing in primary care. *Medical Care, 27,* 478–490. doi:10.1097/00005650-198905000-00004

Hooker, R. S., & McCaig, L. F. (2001). Use of physician assistants and nurse practitioners in primary care, 1995–1999. *Health Affairs, 20,* 231–238. doi:10.1377/hlthaff.20.4.231

Hopewell, A. (2008). First prescribing psychologists in combat theater. *ASAP Tablet,* 9(2), 17–18.

Jaffee, S. R., Harrington, H. L., Cohen, P., & Moffitt, T. E. (2005). Cumulative prevalence of psychiatric disorder in youths. *Journal of the American Academy of Child and Adolescent Psychiatry, 44,* 406–407. doi:10.1097/01.chi.0000155317.38265.61

Kessler, R. C., Demier, O., Frank, R. G., Olfson, M., Pincus, H. A., Walters, E. E., . . . Zaslavsky, A. M. (2005). Prevalence and treatment of mental disorders, 1990 to 2003. *The New England Journal of Medicine, 352,* 2515–2523. doi:10.1056/NEJMsa043266

Krummel, S., & Kathol, R. G. (1987). What you should know about physical evaluations in psychiatric patients: Results of a survey. *General Hospital Psychiatry, 9,* 275–279. doi:10.1016/0163-8343(87)90083-1

Lenz, E. R., Mundinger, M. O., Kane, R. L., Hopkins, S. C., & Lin, S. X. (2004). Primary care outcomes in patients treated by nurse practitioners or physicians: Two-year follow-up. *Medical Care Research and Review, 61*, 332–351. doi:10.1177/1077558704266821

Leon, A. C., Olfson, M., Broadhead, W. E., Barrett, J. E., Blacklow, R. S., Keller, M. B., . . . Weissman, M. M. (1995). Prevalence of mental disorders in primary care. Implications for screening. *Archives of Family Medicine, 4*, 857–861. doi:10.1001/archfami.4.10.857

Linden, M., Lecrubier, Y., Bellantuono, C., Benkert, O., Kisely, S., & Simon, G. (1999). The prescribing of psychotropic drugs by primary care physicians: An international collaborative study. *Journal of Clinical Psychopharmacology, 19*, 132–140. doi:10.1097/00004714-199904000-00007

Massoth, N. A., McGrath, R. E., Bianchi, C., & Singer, J. (1990). Psychologists' attitudes towards prescription privileges. *Professional Psychology, Research and Practice, 21*, 147–149. doi:10.1037/0735-7028.21.2.147

McGrath, R. E. (2008). Prescriptive authority moving forward. *Public Service Psychology: Division 18 Newsletter, 33*(2), pp. 1, 14.

McGrath, R. E., & Muse, M. (2010). Room for a new standard? Response to comments by Heiby. *Journal of Clinical Psychology, 66*, 112–115.

Mechanic, D., McAlpine, D. D., & Rosenthal, M. (2001). Are patients' office visits with physicians getting shorter? *The New England Journal of Medicine, 344*, 198–204. doi:10.1056/NEJM200101183440307

Mojtabai, R., & Olfson, M. (2008). National trends in psychotherapy by office-based psychiatrists. *Archives of General Psychiatry, 65*, 962–970. doi:10.1001/archpsyc.65.8.962

Moore, B. A. (2008). Prescribing psychologists in Iraq: An opportunity for a more comprehensive level of care. *ASAP Tablet, 9*(1), pp. 4, 9.

Mundinger, M. O., Kane, R. L., Lenz, E. R., Totten, A. M., Tsai, W. Y., Cleary, P. D., . . . Shelanski, M. L. (2000). Primary care outcomes in patients treated by nurse practitioners or physicians: A randomized trial. *JAMA, 283*, 59–68. doi:10.1001/jama.283.1.59

Munsey, C. (2006). RxP legislation made historic progress in Hawaii. *Monitor on Psychology, 37*(6), 42.

Muse, M. (2007). Psychology and psychopharmacology. *Papeles del Psicólogo, 28*, 65.

Muse, M., & McGrath, R. E. (2010). Training comparison among three principal professions prescribing psychoactive medications: Psychiatric nurse practitioners, physicians, and medical psychologists. *Journal of Clinical Psychology, 66*, 96–103.

Newman, R., Phelps, R., Sammons, M. T., Dunivin, D. L., & Cullen, E. A. (2000). Evaluation of the Psychopharmacology Demonstration Project: A retrospective analysis. *Professional Psychology, Research and Practice, 31*, 598–603. doi:10.1037/0735-7028.31.6.598

Patterson, C. W. (1978). Psychiatrists and physical examinations: A survey. *The American Journal of Psychiatry, 135*, 967–968.

Pincus, H. A., Tanielian, T. L., Marcus, S. C., Olfson, M., Zarin, D. A., Thompson, J., & Zito, J. M. (1998). Prescribing trends in psychotropic medications: Primary care, psychiatry, and other medical specialties. *JAMA, 279*, 526–531. doi:10.1001/jama.279.7.526

Prescribing psychologist in Iraq awarded Bronze Star medal. (2008). *ASAP Tablet, 9*(2), 5.

Rao, N. R. (2003). Recent trends in psychiatry residency workforce with special reference to international medical graduates. *Academic Psychiatry, 27*, 269–276. doi:10.1176/appi.ap.27.4.269

Richardson, L. A., Keller, A. M., Selby-Harrington, M. L., & Parrish, R. (1996). Identification and treatment of children's mental health problems by primary care providers: A critical review of research. *Archives of Psychiatric Nursing, 10*, 293–303. doi:10.1016/S0883-9417(96)80038-0

Romney, L. (2007, January 6). Prison pay hikes drain staff at state hospitals. *Los Angeles Times*, p. A1.

Sammons, M. T., & Brown, A. B. (1997). The Department of Defense Psychopharmacology Demonstration Project: An evolving program for postdoctoral education in psychology. *Professional Psychology, Research and Practice, 28*, 107–112. doi:10.1037/0735-7028.28.2.107

Sammons, M. T., Gorny, S. W., Zinner, E. S., & Allen, R. P. (2000). Prescriptive authority for psychologists: A consensus of support. *Professional Psychology, Research and Practice, 31*, 604–609. doi:10.1037/0735-7028.31.6.604

Sammons, M. T., & Schmidt, N. B. (Eds.). (2003). *Combined treatments for mental disorders: A guide to psychological and pharmacological interventions*. Washington, DC: American Psychological Association.

Speer, A., & Bess, D. T. (2003). Evaluation of compensation of nonphysician providers. *American Journal of Health-System Pharmacy, 60*, 78–80.

St-Pierre, E. S., & Melnyk, W. T. (2004). The prescription privilege debate in Canada: The voices of today's and tomorrow's psychologists. *Canadian Psychology, 45*, 284–292. doi:10.1037/h0086999

U.S. Congress, Office of Technology Assessment. (1986). *Nurse practitioners, physician assistants, and certified nurse-midwives: A policy analysis* (Health Technology Case Study 37, OTA-HCS-37). Washington, DC: U.S. Government Printing Office.

U.S. General Accounting Office. (1997). *Defense health care: Need for more prescribing psychologists is NOT adequately justified* (GAO/HEHS-97-83). Washington, DC: Author.

U.S. General Accounting Office. (1999). *Prescribing psychologists: DOD Demonstration participants perform well but have effect on readiness or costs* (GAO/HEHS-99-98). Washington, DC: Author.

van der Waals, F. W., Mohrs, J., & Foet, M. (1993). Sex differences among recipients of benzodiazepines in Dutch general practice. *British Medical Journal, 307,* 363–366. doi:10.1136/bmj.307.6900.363

Vector Research. (1996). *Cost-effectiveness and feasibility of the DoD Psychopharmacology Demonstration Project: Final report.* Arlington, VA: Author.

Walkup, J. T., Albano, A. M., Piacentini, J., Birmaher, B., Compton, S. N. Sherrill, J. T., et al. (2008). Cognitive behavioral therapy, sertraline, or a combination in childhood anxiety. *The New England Journal of Medicine, 359.* doi:10.1056/NEJMoa0804633.

Walters, G. D. (2001). A meta-analysis of opinion data on the prescription privilege debate. *Canadian Psychology, 42,* 119–125. doi:10.1037/h0086886

Wang, P. S., Demler, O., Olfson, M., Pincus, H. A., Wells, K. B., & Kessler, R. C. (2006). Changing profiles of service sectors used for mental health care in the United States. *The American Journal of Psychiatry, 163,* 1187–1198. doi:10.1176/appi.ajp.163.7.1187

Wiggins, J. G., & Cummings, N. A. (1998). National study of the experience of psychologists with psychotropic medication and psychotherapy. *Professional Psychology, Research and Practice, 29,* 549–552. doi:10.1037/0735-7028.29.6.549

Wiggins, J. G., & Wedding, D. (2004). Prescribing, professional identity, and cost. *Professional Psychology, Research and Practice, 35,* 148–150. doi:10.1037/0735-7028.35.2.148

Williams-Russo, P. (1996). Barriers to diagnosis and treatment of depression in primary care settings. *The American Journal of Geriatric Psychiatry, 4,* S84–S90.

Younger, R. D. (2007a). Enhanced practice psychology on the front lines: Personal coping in war. *ASAP Tablet, 8*(4), 4.

Younger, R. D. (2007b). From the front lines of psychologists prescribing: A MASH case. *ASAP Tablet, 8*(3), 4.

2

THE EVOLUTION OF TRAINING GUIDELINES IN PHARMACOTHERAPY FOR PSYCHOLOGISTS

LINDA F. CAMPBELL AND RONALD FOX

Education and training in psychopharmacology for prescriptive authority is an endeavor that has evolved over the past 2 decades to meet the continually changing professional landscape for psychologists. Psychopharmacological education and training encompasses fundamental domains of psychology, such as the teaching of basic neuroscience, adherence to ethical behavior, valuing of diversity, identity within a scientist–practitioner model, and a commitment to quality assurance. It is also true, however, that psychopharmacological education and training represent a distinct and significant expansion in the scope of practice in psychology. Extraordinary challenges, intense debate, high-stakes decision making, and grappling with new questions that have yet to be answered characterize this journey.

This chapter (a) reviews the roots of early curriculum development, (b) discusses the foundational principles of the American Psychological Association's (APA) 1996 *Recommended Postdoctoral Training in Psychopharmacology for Prescription Privileges* and inherent problems that prompted the need for revision, (c) describes the 2009 *Recommended Postdoctoral Education and Training Program in Psychopharmacology for Prescriptive Authority* and key features of the revision, and (d) explains the 2009 *Designation Criteria for Education and Training Programs in Preparation for Prescriptive Authority*.

HISTORICAL ROOTS

The debate over psychologists having prescriptive authority began in the early 1990s. Those who saw either the desirability or inevitability of the role of psychotropic medications in the treatment of psychological disorders moved the debate from discussion to action in less than a decade (Brentar & McNamara, 1991; Burns, DeLeon, Chemtob, Welch, & Samuels, 1988; DeLeon, Folen, Jennings, Willis, & Wright, 1991; DeLeon, Fox, & Graham, 1991; Fox, 1988a, 1988b). Fundamentally important steps were taken by several groups of psychologists who organized to move the prescriptive authority agenda forward. Even though there were differences among the initial activists, all agreed on two observations: (a) psychologists would need specific and additional training beyond the current doctoral-training program requirements and (b) a curriculum would need to be developed that included content from other health service prescribing professions but also would be specifically designed for psychologists and psychological practice.

Each of these initiatives made principle and distinct contributions to the research on the state of psychotropic medications, identification of relevant training models in other professions, and the understanding of the pedagogical and practical variables within the profession necessary to evaluate the curricular needs and potential training structures. These foundational initiatives and their unique contributions are described here.

1992 Proposed Curriculum for Psychopharmacology Training for Professional Psychologists

This early model curriculum, developed by Fox, Schwelitz, and Barclay (1992), became the blueprint for the continued development and subsequent iterations of curricular models and remains today the foundation of the 1996 and 2009 APA model curricula. The Fox et al. (1992) curriculum has withstood the test of time, and even through several subsequent revisions this curriculum sufficiently captures the essential specialty domains necessary for psychopharmacological training. The curriculum included courses in biochemistry, psychopharmacology, physiology and drug interactions, psychopharmacology, clinical psychopharmacology and therapeutics, ethics issues, clinical pharmacology laboratory, chemical dependency, neuropsychology and laboratory, and psychopathology, for a total of 39 academic quarter hours (390 class hours). It also identified two necessary components of training that would be challenges and, in fact, continue to be so: (a) Required human and financial resources would be substantial, and the faculty expertise in existing doctoral-training programs would not be adequate; and (b) supervised practica would be an essential component of quality training, but several obstacles would have to be overcome to make such practica possible.

Report of the Ad Hoc Task Force on Psychopharmacology of the American Psychological Association (Smyer et al., 1993)

In 1990, the APA Board of Directors authorized an ad hoc task force charged with evaluating the factors involved in pursuing prescription privileges for psychologists. The charge was to determine training criteria that ensured competent practice and to develop the commensurate curriculum models to accomplish the training goals. The summary findings of this task force were presented in the *Report of the Ad Hoc Task Force on Psychopharmacology* (Smyer et al., 1993). Four of the recommendations that emanate from this report became major contributions to curriculum development and program design. Two of the important curricular contributions were the (a) proposal for three levels of training and (b) postdoctoral or internship level training for supervised practicum experiences. The first reflected the realization that psychologists would vary in the level of competence they hope to achieve as psychopharmacologists in light of their professional roles. The task force recommended three levels of training that would accomplish the competency expectations:

- Level 1: Basic psychopharmacology education would result in requisite knowledge of the biological bases and mechanisms by which drugs affect the neurotransmitter systems. This training would be acquired through a separate survey course in psychopharmacology at the graduate level.
- Level 2: Collaborative practice (consultation-liaison model) would build on Level 1 and would reflect the knowledge base for collaboration in managing medications prescribed for mental disorders by other professionals. Psychologists with Level 2 training would then be able to integrate collaborating medication management into psychosocial treatments but were not expected to prescribe.
- Level 3: Prescription privileges would prepare psychologists for independent practice, limited only by scope of practice, as are other professions (e.g., dentists, optometrists, nurse practitioners).

The second major curricular contribution of the task force was the specific recommendation for supervised practice, either during an expanded internship or a residency during a postdoctoral year. A supervised practicum or clinical experience became an essential component of training but also a most challenging one to accomplish.

The ad hoc task force also made two important recommendations for a more comprehensive program model: (a) The task force realized that Level 3 could not feasibly be matriculated through traditional continuing education and recommended a certificate program that would allow licensed, doctoral-level psychologists to engage in training; and (b) the task force foresaw the importance of selective and specific use of traditional continuing education for levels of psychopharmacological training. Continuing education was envisioned as appropriate for continued learning for Level 1 after a basic psychopharmacology course, appropriate for Level 2 after advanced training, and not likely to be feasible for Level 3. Finally, the description of content domains provided in the report remained consistent with Fox et al. (1992).

Report of the Blue Ribbon Panel—Professional Education Task Force of the California Psychological Association and the California School of Professional Psychology (1995)—Los Angeles

The Blue Ribbon Panel was funded by the APA Committee for the Advancement of Professional Practice (CAPP). The task force was charged with (a) reviewing curricula used by other health professions in teaching prescription of medication, (b) incorporating gender and cultural sensitivity into training, and (c) drafting recommended requirements for training psychologists to prescribe medications. The Blue Ribbon Panel was chaired by Ronald Fox and included psychologists (some of whom had been trained to prescribe) and several physicians. The panel made several recommendations that have guided the evolving framework of psychopharmacological training. First, the psychosocial model of prescription for psychologists rests heavily on the importance of prescription decisions happening within the context of the assessment of the whole person. Age, gender, ethnicity, race, disability, and other diversity factors have been virtually overlooked in many health treatment environments. The psychological model of prescriptive authority adds prescribing as an ancillary skill to traditional practices rather than as a replacement for psychological practices. Second, the curriculum blueprint developed by Fox et al. (1992) and advanced by the APA Ad Hoc Task Force (Smyer et al., 1993) became foundational didactic content for the Blue Ribbon recommended curriculum. This curriculum in turn provided the basis for the APA 1996 *Recommended Postdoctoral Training in Psychopharmacology for Prescription Privileges*.

The findings of the Blue Ribbon Panel also advanced the development of psychopharmacological training for psychologists in that subsequent training criteria have been consistent with the panel's recommendations:

- The coursework should lead to a prescribing proficiency. In fact, prescription has been classified by the APA Commission on Specialties and Proficiencies as a proficiency.

- The training program would be postdoctoral and even post-licensure as a psychologist. This requirement became part of the criteria for training in the 1996 APA Model Curriculum.
- A supervised practicum of 100 patients conducted in inpatient and outpatient settings with a balance to diagnostic mix was also incorporated into the 1996 APA model.
- The range of contact hours was identified as 260 to 435 for didactic work and approximately 18 months for the practicum.
- The recommendations were designed to lead to a certificate of proficiency for doctoral-level psychologists. In fact, as the credentialing process has progressed, certificates of proficiency and masters degrees have both been awarded.

Final Report of the Board of Educational Affairs (BEA) Working Group to Develop a Level 1 Curriculum for Psychopharmacology Education and Training (APA, 1995)

The 1992 report of the APA ad hoc task force on psychopharmacology calling for development of three levels of training, described earlier in this chapter, resulted in the formation of a BEA working group that developed both Levels 1 and 2. Level 1 as recommended is a basic course in clinical psychopharmacology. The modules include the following: (1) biological bases of psychopharmacological treatment, (2–3) principles of psychopharmacological treatment, (4) general introduction to clinical psychopharmacology, (5) treatment of psychoactive substance use disorders, (6) treatment of psychotic disorders, (7) treatment of mood disorders, (8) treatment of anxiety disorders, and (9) treatment of developmental disorders.

Final Report of the Board of Educational Affairs (BEA) Working Group to Develop Curriculum for Level 2 Training in Psychopharmacology (APA, 1997)

The BEA working group also developed a Level 2 curriculum that involved advanced knowledge of psychodiagnostics, physical assessment, physical function tests, and drug interactions important for particular populations or chronic disorders. As in the development of Level 1, the working group developed stand-alone modules for adaptability to various settings. The training is viewed as postdoctoral, and therefore the format lends itself to psychologists who may subsequently seek prescriptive authority. The modules are designed for use with (a) children–adolescents, (b) older adults, (c) adults with serious mental illness, and (d) mental retardation and developmental disabilities.

1996 RECOMMENDED POSTDOCTORAL TRAINING IN PSYCHOPHARMACOLOGY FOR PRESCRIPTION PRIVILEGES

The development and adoption of an APA-recommended postdoctoral curriculum was an important and exciting event in the evolution of prescriptive authority for psychologists. This document, approved by the APA Council of Representatives in August 1996, provided the road map for the profession in terms of course of training and legislation.

The curriculum was developed to ensure quality, clarify the expectations of trainees and the programs, and be adaptable to those trainees at differing points in their careers and levels of expertise. The program of didactic courses and clinical practica were expected to be an organized, systematic, and sequential course of study rather than individually selected learning experiences. Some of the key features included the following:

- The model postdoctoral training program rested upon a psychosocial model, not a medical model. This foundational concept is most important in understanding the values and goals of psychologists as prescribers. Professional ethics, respect for the welfare of others, beneficence, and awareness of those with diverse characteristics (e.g., age, ethnicity, gender, race, disability) are critically important factors in prescribing yet are often ignored. The authority to withdraw a patient from medication is as important as putting a patient on medication. The reciprocal interaction of physical health and mental health is irrefutable. Psychologists understand this importance between treatment of brain disorders and psychological treatment.
- The model postdoctoral training program assumed a scientist–practitioner model. Psychologists are committed to the scientific method and the knowledge base that results from scientific endeavors. Psychologists will not be prescribing practitioners only, but they will also contribute to the expanding knowledge base and scientific advancement in psychopharmacology.
- The model postdoctoral-training program required applicants to have a doctoral degree and to be licensed. This model builds on the competencies that are reflected by the training completed in the doctoral program and internship. For example, the curriculum assumes students have had numerous experiences in making ethical decisions and interpreting the laws and regulations of their jurisdictions. If this knowledge base could not be assumed, then advanced-level ethical concepts or clinical experiences assumed in the curriculum would not have an adequate foundation. A licensed psychologist has at the very least completed an

internship, possibly a postdoctoral experience, and some practice. These clinical experiences give psychologists a competency base from which to make decisions and to take action. The same readiness principle can be cited for issues that surround diversity, theory, leadership, and advocacy that need to be addressed in the training.

- A clinical practicum or supervised clinical experience was considered by all working groups that have contributed to the evolution of the curriculum as one of the most important and central components of training. The practicum was given parameters, including number of patients, patient mix that is consistent with current and expected future practice of the psychologist, type of settings, and quality of supervision.

- The model postdoctoral-training program was required to be offered within a regionally accredited institution of higher learning or another appropriately accredited provider. This requirement was adopted to maintain quality assurance.

Training Curriculum

The required didactic instruction of a minimum of 300 contact hours included the following core content areas: (a) the neurosciences, (b) pharmacology and psychopharmacology, (c) physiology and pathophysiology, (d) physical and laboratory assessment, and (e) clinical pharmacotherapeutics. Table 2.1 shows the recommended contact hours in each area (note that these summed to 350 hr). Clinical practicum included the following contact hours: (a) a minimum of 100 patients seen for medication, (b) inpatient and outpatient placements, (c) inclusion of appropriate didactic instruction, and (d) a minimum of 2 hr weekly of individual supervision.

The Need for Revision

The development and approval of the *Recommended Postdoctoral Training in Psychopharmacology for Prescription Privileges* (APA, 1996) was critically important to psychology for several reasons. The credibility of training programs was directly connected to adoption of an approved curriculum. The willingness of psychologists–trainees to matriculate through a program was dependent on the trainees believing that their educational experience would be of assured quality. Psychologists who were promoting prescriptive authority legislation needed to have a bona fide curriculum to refute negative characterizations of psychologists' legislative goals. The model curriculum has served a vital purpose at an important time in the development of this

TABLE 2.1
1996 Model Curriculum Contact Hours

Topic	Hours
Neurosciences	
Neuroanatomy	25
Neurophysiology	25
Neurolochemistry	25
Clinical and research pharmacology and psychopharmacology	
Pharmacology	30
Clinical pharmacology	30
Psychopharmacology	45
Development psychopharmacology	10
Chemical dependency and chronic pain management	15
Pathophysiology	60
Introduction to physical assessment and laboratory exams	45
Pharmacotherapeutics	
Professional, ethical, and legal issues	15
Psychotherapy/pharmacotherapy interactions	10
Computer-based aids to practice	5
Pharmacoepidemiology	10

Note. Data from *Recommended postdoctoral training in psychopharmacology for prescription privileges* (APA, 1996).

initiative. However, the model came due for 10-year review in 2006, as is APA policy. Additionally, attempts to implement the model curriculum generated dissatisfaction with impractical elements of the model after several years. The primary concerns that represented an impetus for revision were the following:

- Clinical practicum: The logistical structure of supervised practice, the politics of supervision, access to patients, and human resources were reasons that the clinical practicum was most difficult to accomplish. In psychology doctoral practica and internships, as in psychopharmacology practica, students are not licensed to practice but can practice under the supervision of a licensed psychologist because the practice of psychology is within legal scope of practice. In psychopharmacology, the psychologist–trainee is not licensed for prescribing. This meant that physicians and other licensed professionals had to serve as supervisors, and most were reluctant to supervise what could be interpreted as illegal practice. The politics of psychologists who were expanding their scope of practice to encompass prescriptive authority created very organized and well-financed opposition from medicine. Those with credentials to qualify as supervisors were part of the medical community and were reluctant to participate. Until there are more prescribing psychologists who can supervise trainees, the supervision of psychologists–trainees is untenable in many geographical areas. As a result, the programs were not able to incorporate practicum into the didactic training program successfully. Finally, programs did not have the human resources in credentialed faculty to do the supervision in house.

- Continuing education (CE): There were limited means through which psychologists could acquire the psychopharmacology training because there were so few organized, systematic, and sequenced training programs. Moreover, after the approval of the 1996 Postdoctoral Training Model, the APA Continuing Education Committee was asked to oversee the development and dissemination of a curriculum based on the newly approved criteria and outline for coursework. At the time, it was also considered a possibility that the materials developed might be used in providing organized programs of continuing education. Individual psychologists who wanted to acquire the training but did not have access to organized and sequenced programs advocated for a continuing education route to matriculating the prescribing curriculum. Over several years of discussion about the potential role of continuing education in psychopharmacology training, the APA Continuing Education Committee, which is charged with approval of organizations as sponsors of CE for psychologists, reiterated at their February 2004 policy meeting that their review does not encompass specific content of the programs offered by sponsors, nor are the CE participants evaluated in any way for competency or skill acquisition in the content material. The Continuing Education Committee also rejected a proposal to develop a role in the credentialing process for individual psychopharmacology students on the grounds that such oversight would be outside the scope of responsibilities and capabilities of the committee.

- Regionally accredited institution requirement: This requirement was viewed as unfairly excluding potential training institutions that were not regionally accredited and essentially giving universities exclusive rights to the training. On the other hand, the regional accreditation requirement was viewed by many who were concerned about quality assurance as the safety net in avoiding exploitation of trainees.

2009 RECOMMENDED POSTDOCTORAL EDUCATION AND TRAINING PROGRAM IN PSYCHOPHARMACOLOGY FOR PRESCRIPTIVE AUTHORITY

The 2009 *Recommended Postdoctoral Education and Training Program in Psychopharmacology for Prescriptive Authority* (APA, 2009b; see Exhibit 2.1) was initially and primarily focused on resolving the difficulties evidenced in the 1996 recommended postdoctoral-training model. The change in terminology from *prescription privileges* to *prescriptive authority* in itself reflects the maturing of psychologists' understanding of terminology appropriate to prescribing and serves as a metaphor for increasing sophistication that surrounds the pragmatics of prescribing. Additionally, the title revision reflects the greater focus on not only education (i.e., curriculum) but also on the training program itself as the focus for quality assurance elements. The APA task force charged with the revision also realized that a major conceptual shift was necessary in the revision of the model to accommodate other evolving concepts in the profession, such as the movement toward competency-based evaluation (APA, 2006a). The profession of psychology, other health professions, educational technology, and the state of health care itself had dramatically changed over the 10-year period so that the task was to create a new framework that would maximize the potential for success of psychopharmacology practiced by psychologists. The 2009 recommended postdoctoral education and training model was originally approved in principle at the August 2007 Council of Representatives meeting, pending development of some sort of quality control mechanism for such programs. It was given full approval at the 2009 August Council meeting along with the approval of the 2009 designation system that addressed this quality control issue.

Resolutions to the 1996 Postdoctoral Training Challenges

The 1996 model was adopted when there were only a few programs and no enacted legislation. The challenges that emerged during the subsequent 10 years were natural outcomes of the evolving field and the difficulties that emerged in implementing a new scope of practice. Several challenges in the 1996 postdoctoral training model were identified for program revision with the following being the most prominent.

Supervised Clinical Experience

The 1996 program term *practicum* has been replaced with the term *supervised clinical experience*, which more aptly describes the integrated nature of the clinical experience in this model. Rather than being a separate and final requirement, the supervised clinical experience may be integrated into

EXHIBIT 2.1
2009 Model Curriculum

Didactic Content Areas

Basic science
  Anatomy and physiology
  Biochemistry
Neurosciences
  Neuroanatomy
  Neurophysiology
  Neurochemistry
Physical assessment and laboratory exams
  Physical assessment
  Laboratory and radiological assessment
  Medical terminology and documentation
Clinical medicine and pathophysiology
  Pathophysiology with particular emphasis on cardiac, renal, hepatic, neurologic,
    gastrointestinal, hematologic, dermatologic, and endocrine systems
  Clinical medicine with particular emphasis on signs, symptoms and treatment
    of disease states with behavioral, cognitive and emotional manifestations
    or comorbidities
  Differential diagnosis
  Clinical correlations: illustration of the content of this domain through case study
  Substance-related and co-occuring disorders
  Chronic pain management
Clinical and research pharmacology and psychopharmacology
  Pharmacology
  Clinical pharmacology
  Pharmacogenetics
  Psychopharmacology
  Developmental psychopharmacology
  Issues of diversity in pharmacological practice
Clinical pharmacotherapeutics
  Combined therapies: psychotherapy/pharmacotherapy interactions
  Computer-based aids to practice
  Pharmacoepidemiology
Research
  Methodology and design of psychopharmacological research
  Interpretation and evaluation of research
  U.S. Food and Drug Administration drug development and other regulatory
    processes
Professional, ethical, and legal issues
  Application of existing law, standards and guidelines to pharmacological practice
  Relationships with pharmaceutical industry
    Conflict of interest
    Evaluation of pharmaceutical marketing practices
    Critical consumer
Supervised Clinical Experience
  Physical exam and mental status
  Review of systems
  Medical history interview and documentation
  Assessment: Indications and interpretation
  Differential diagnosis
  Integrated treatment planning
  Consultation and collaboration
  Treatment management

Note. Data from *Recommended postdoctoral education and training program in psychopharmacology for prescriptive authority* (APA, 2009b).

the didactic coursework or continue to be completed separately. The purpose of the supervised clinical experience is to (a) provide ongoing integration of didactic and applied clinical knowledge throughout the learning sequence, and (b) facilitate both formative and summative assessment of competency in skills and applied knowledge (APA, 2009a). The integration of clinical experience with coursework facilitates the application of the concepts acquired through the coursework. The supervised clinical experience requirement may be met in a variety of ways that include the use of emerging technology and that allow evaluation of competency through other means in addition to face-to-face contact. The supervised clinical experience is evaluated by assessing achieved competencies.

Program Evaluation

The postdoctoral education and training program as an organized and sequential program of instruction at the postdoctoral level is a foundational concept on which the program is built. The use of CE as a means of evaluation of individuals and quality assurance of programs was not tenable. The CE structure within APA was capable of evaluating neither individual students' progress nor the effectiveness of training programs. Psychopharmacology is recognized by APA as a proficiency (APA, 2005), and proficiencies are not eligible under APA guidelines for accreditation consideration. Instead, a designation system was proposed as the appropriate mechanism for quality assurance of training programs in proficiencies. A designation system evaluates whether programs meet the standards established for those programs seeking designation status. Consequently, the model called for a designation system to achieve quality assurance.

Regionally Accredited Institutions

Regional accreditation does provide an alternative route to ensuring quality. However, it was recognized that other organizations could achieve the expected level of quality and yet not be able to be regionally accredited. For the field to grow, it became evident that an alternative means of program evaluation was necessary. The designation process and the competency-based evaluation methods can be most effective in providing oversight of program quality.

Essential Elements of the 2009 Model Postdoctoral Education and Training Program

The 2009 Postdoctoral Education and Training Model Program is assuredly a revision of the 1996 Postdoctoral Training Model Program; however, the program characteristics and the process of matriculation are reconceptualized to better meet the learning needs of trainees who are using advances in educational technology and competency-based assessment.

Postdoctoral Education and Training

The 2009 training model is designed to be a postdoctoral program. The program is an organized, sequential, and integrated advanced training experience. The coursework, integration of clinical experience and didactic courses, and knowledge and skills gained in a doctoral training program are assumed. The 2009 model retained the prerequisites of the 1996 model in requirements for matriculation: (a) a doctoral degree in psychology, (b) current licensure as a psychologist, and (c) practice as a health services provider as defined by one's jurisdictional law. However, where the 1996 model also listed prerequisite basic science and neuroscience courses, those are now included in the curriculum and can be transferred in for up to 20% of the curriculum. This standard allows basic science and neuroscience to be taught in other programs, including doctoral level programs. The limit of 20% allows the training program to meet the spirit and the standard of an organized, sequential, and integrated postdoctoral psychopharmacology program.

Integrated Didactic Instruction and Supervised Clinical Experience

The supervised clinical experience was described earlier, but it must be mentioned again as an essential element. The integrated nature of the didactic instruction and the supervised clinical experience allow trainees to implement conceptual knowledge and assimilate new skills through application. This method of integrating didactic instruction and supervised clinical experience is described in the didactic content section of the 2009 document. Use of technology and new learning methods are cited (e.g., problem-based learning, computerized patients; simulations using layered decision models, and skills-based demonstrations; APA, 2009a) as means of advancing the integration of knowledge acquisition and application. It is interesting to note that the didactic curriculum is largely unchanged from the initial course content of the Blue Ribbon Panel. The supervised clinical experience should be an organized sequence of training that is reflective of the didactic content and the totality of the program.

Elements of a Competency Model

Education and training programs, particularly in health professions and other practice professions, have been adopting competency-based methods of evaluation for some years. Most educators would agree that assessing competency rather than fulfilling number of courses or hours is more effective for ensuring a level of skill and knowledge that a training program expects and requires. The competency model, however, is a significant departure from traditional evaluation methods. For this reason, the 2009 model is a hybrid model that mixes competency (e.g., in the supervised clinical experience) and traditional evaluation (e.g., contact hour requirements for didactic coursework). The development of educational learning experiences is in a developmental stage in psychology. For a period of time, training programs in psychopharmacology, in general doctoral training, and other educational experiences will be mixed models that move into greater preparation and capability for competency training and evaluation. The APA Task Force on the Assessment of Competence in Professional Psychology developed 15 principles that are a useful resource (APA, 2006b).

Education and Training in Issues of Diversity

Inherent in the development of psychopharmacological training for psychologists is the value and importance of the psychosocial model of practice. An integral part of this model is the responsibility to understand the many factors that affect the health behaviors and quality of life of patients, especially issues of diversity. The APA (2002) *Ethical Principles of Psychologists and Code of Conduct* reflects the profession's commitment to the welfare of patients and the responsibility of psychologists to be competent in treating diverse populations. Prescriptive authority grants psychologists an opportunity to practice their integrated profession in a holistic manner not before possible.

Lifelong Learning

Postdoctoral training programs in psychopharmacology will prepare psychologists for skilled and competent practice. The development of new medications, advances in technology, and biomedical research findings will require dedication to continued learning throughout the life span. Postdoctoral training programs in psychopharmacology will prepare psychologists not only to analyze and interpret scientific findings but also to engage in the scientific method themselves and to be participants in the pursuit of advances in their domain.

2009 DESIGNATION CRITERIA FOR EDUCATION AND TRAINING PROGRAMS IN PREPARATION FOR PRESCRIPTIVE AUTHORITY

Training programs typically exist within institutions in which the program is accredited, the university is regionally accredited, or in which another credential is widely recognized for quality assurance. These are methods by which potential students may know that programs meet the requirements for which the program claims. When the 2009 revision of the training model removed the requirement of regional accreditation, another form of oversight and verification of standards was needed. Several factors contributed to the need for a mechanism to ensure that programs provide the quality and standard of training experience delineated in the Recommended Postdoctoral Education and Training Program: (a) the movement toward a competency-based model, (b) a breadth of formats in which programs matriculate, and (c) the integration of didactic content and supervised clinical experience (APA, 2008). The designation program document was presented and approved by the APA Council of Representatives at the August 2009 meeting.

The composition of the designation body needed to be representative of the groups of interest and expertise in psychopharmacology while avoiding conflict of interest. Currently, those representative groups are psychopharmacology education and training programs, relevant basic scientists, educators, relevant public interests representatives, and practitioners.

It is important to note that training programs need to be recognizable as an organized, integrated sequence of study and experience. In support of this principle, designated programs are expected to have an identifiable organization, curriculum, and faculty (APA, 2008). The designation criteria defined and described in that document delineate three major components, all of which have been discussed in this chapter: (a) essential elements, (b) the program characteristics, and (c) the didactic curriculum and supervised clinical experience. The essential elements were highlighted in the document in order to make transparent the major revisions from the 1996 document. Curricular and program standards are integrally linked in that the quality of the curriculum can only be maintained through the framework of high-quality program administration. The task force developed the designation criteria to be congruent with the curriculum–clinical experience and program standards. Education and training programs additionally must be mindful of the quality of learning experience provided to students and the importance of creating and maintaining a healthy, ethical, and professional learning environment. With these priorities in mind, the task force addressed these three components of designation: (a) program characteristics, (b) curriculum, and (c) students. The designation format identifies standards in each of these three classifications and a method for documentation.

Program Characteristics

The criteria identified to evaluate program characteristics convey the importance of applicant programs evidencing sufficient resources, sustainability, and an appropriate learning environment. Program criteria and requisite documentation were developed to most effectively facilitate understanding designation expectations of the designation process.

Ways in which programs may demonstrate adherence to standards include

- evidence of doctoral program completion and licensure in meeting admissions standards;
- program stance on transfer credit through publicly available policy statements;
- citation of the Ethics Code in policy statements, admissions materials, and student handbook materials for adherence to the APA Ethics Code and intent to abide by the Ethics Code;
- publicly available materials, mission statement, and program description for transparency to the public;
- financial resources demonstrated through financial reports and budgetary documents and physical resources through library materials, facility and laboratory sites, and electronic resources;
- description of organizational structure and qualifications of administrators for evidence of governance ability;
- provision of curriculum vitas, course syllabi, and other professional credentials for faculty skills and competence;
- evidence of appropriate contractual agreements and means of evaluating supervisor competence in assessing quality assurance; and
- description of procedures for program evaluation and maintenance of current teaching materials for program self-evaluation.

A documentation section accompanies the elaboration of each program criterion and explains how the programs may meet standards.

Curriculum

The education and training of psychologists occurs within a program that reflects the recommended didactic curriculum and supervised experience. Program resources are available for stability of funding and continuity of faculty in facilitating opportunities to teach, supervise, and evaluate students (APA, 2008).

Programs offer an organized sequential course of study that reflects the recommended curriculum and supervised clinical experiences as evidenced through the following: (a) an organized sequence of courses with documentation from syllabi; (b) frequent evaluation of students' knowledge, application of that knowledge, and feedback to the students; (c) periodic program evaluation of a self study or external review method; and (d) a certification method, documenting the students' completion of the program (APA, 2008).

Designation evaluation of curriculum could be evidenced by syllabi for didactic courses; however, evaluation of clinical experience is a more difficult task. The documentation section provides a grid for recording the intersection of supervised clinical experiences with various didactic experiences and simplifies the means by which individualized integrated experiences may be logged. There is also a capstone experience required that involves integration of the knowledge, skills, and attitudes psychologists are expected to master during matriculation. To receive the certificate of completion, students must successfully finish the didactic and experiential requirements as well as the capstone experience within 5 years.

Students

Designation perspectives on engagement with students include criteria that clarify expectations of psychologist–students (e.g., licensure, active enrollment) and identify expectations of faculty and the program (e.g., proper maintenance of student records, provision of due process). The designation document supports the admissions requirement that all applicants be doctoral-level licensed psychologists. This requirement is in keeping with the premise of building on the doctoral program and incorporating knowledge and skills from that training into advanced competencies in the psychopharmacology program.

Programs that achieve designation status are committed to demonstrating fair and just treatment of diverse populations of students and are prepared to report the number of students enrolled, whether they are active students, and the length of time toward graduation. Additionally, student records, due process, and assurance of continued licensure are reviewed.

CONCLUSION

The 1996 and 2009 APA Recommended Postdoctoral Education and Training Programs and the efforts of those in leadership advanced psychology significantly into the health care arena. The biopsychosocial model of practice espoused by psychology will become a reality as prescriptive authority is achieved within the profession. Psychologists will be able to incorporate medication evaluation with contemporary practices of psychology to treat the whole person and to provide a much richer treatment for our patients–clients.

REFERENCES

American Psychological Association. (1995). *Final report of the BEA working group to develop a level 1 curriculum for psychopharmacology education and training.* Washington, DC: Author.

American Psychological Association. (1996). *Recommended postdoctoral training in psychopharmacology for prescription privileges.* Washington, DC: Author.

American Psychological Association. (1997). *Curriculum for level 2 training in psychopharmacology.* Washington, DC: Author.

American Psychological Association. (2002). *Ethical principles of psychologists and code of conduct.* Washington, DC: Author.

American Psychological Association. (2005). *Report of the BEA task force on quality assurance of education and training for recognized proficiencies of professional psychology.* Washington, DC: Author.

American Psychological Association. (2006a). *Recommended postdoctoral education and training programs in psychopharmacology for prescriptive authority.* Washington, DC: Author.

American Psychological Association. (2006b). *Report of the AP Task Force on the assessment of competence in professional psychology* (pp. 3–7). Washington, DC: Author.

American Psychological Association. (2008). *Designation criteria for education and training programs in preparation for prescriptive authority.* Washington, DC: Author.

American Psychological Association. (2009a). *Designation criteria for education and training programs in preparation for prescriptive authority.* Retrieved from http://www.apa.org/about/governance/council/policy/rxp-model-curriculum.pdf

American Psychological Association. (2009b). *Recommended postdoctoral education and training program in psychopharmacology for prescriptive authority.* Retrieved from http://www.apa.org/about/governance/council/policy/rxp-model-curriculum.pdf

Brentar, J., & McNamara, J. (1991). The right to prescribe medication: Considerations for professional psychology. *Professional Psychology: Research and Practice, 22,* 179–187.

Burns, S. M., DeLeon, P. H., Chemtob, C. M., Welch, B. L., & Samuels, R.M. (1988). Psychotropic medication: A new techniques for psychology? *Psychotherapy Theory: Research, Practice, and Training, 25,* 508–515.

DeLeon, P. H., Folen, R. A., Jennings, F. L., Willis, D. J., & Wright, R. H. (1991). The case for prescription privileges: A logical evolution of professional practice. *Journal of Clinical Child Psychology, 20,* 254–267.

DeLeon, P. H., Fox, R. E., & Graham, S. R. (1991). Prescription privileges: Psychology's next frontier? *American Psychologist, 46,* 384–393.

Fox, R. E., (1988a). Prescription privileges: Their implications for the practice of psychology. *Psychotherapy, 25,* 501–507.

Fox, R. E. (1988b). Some practical and legal objections to prescription privileges for psychologists. *Psychotherapy in Private Practice, 6,* 23–30.

Fox, R. E., Schwelitz, F. D., & Barclay, A. G. (1992). A proposed curriculum for psychopharmacology training for professional psychologists. *Professional Psychology: Research and Practice, 23,* 216–219. doi:10.1037/0735-7028.23.3.216

Professional Education Task Force of the California Psychological Association and the California School of Professional Psychology. (1995). *Report of the blue ribbon panel.* Blue Ribbon. Unpublished manuscript.

Smyer, M. A., Balster, R. L., Egli, D., Johnson, D. I., Kilbey, M. M., Leith, N. J., & Puente, A. E. (1993). Summary of the report of the Ad Hoc Task Force on Psychopharmacology of the American Psychological Association. *Professional Psychology: Research and Practice, 24,* 394–403. doi:10.1037/0735-7028.24.4.394

3

THE PSYCHOPHARMACOLOGY DEMONSTRATION PROJECT: WHAT DID IT TEACH US, AND WHERE ARE WE NOW?

MORGAN T. SAMMONS

The Department of Defense (DOD) Psychopharmacology Demonstration Project (PDP), which trained 10 psychologists to become independent prescribers of psychotropic medications, ran between the years of 1991 and 1997. It has been rather exhaustively described elsewhere (e.g., DeLeon, Folen, Jennings, Willis, & Wright, 1991; DeLeon, Fox, & Graham, 1991; DeLeon, Sammons, & Sexton, 1995; Dunivin & Orabona, 1999; Laskow & Grill, 2003; Newman, Phelps, Sammons, Dunivin, & Cullen, 2000; Sammons & Brown, 1997; Sammons, Sexton, & Meredith, 1996), so the purpose of this chapter will not be to recreate a history of the PDP but to point to lessons that can be acquired from that history and to underscore the extent to which political and guild interests shaped the curriculum of that program as well as how it has influenced prescribing psychology in the military. This chapter is written from the perspective of one of the original participants in that program who has subsequently followed the prescriptive authority movement with keen interest.

The PDP was perhaps one of the most controversial initiatives undertaken by psychologists in the public or private sector. Opposition from other professional guilds was the source of most of the controversy. It has perhaps been forgotten that the medical and psychiatric establishments played a key role in both developing and evaluating the curriculum of the PDP. The Blue

Ribbon Panel convened by the U.S. Army Surgeon General to recommend suggested curricula was composed of members of the American Medical Association (AMA), the American Psychiatric Association, and the American College of Neuropsychopharmacology (ACNP) in addition to representatives from the American Psychological Association (APA). The AMA, the American Psychiatric Association, and the ACNP all took pains to explicitly express their opposition to the project (unpublished memorandum, Deputy Surgeon General of the Army, "Update of limited prescription privileges training for DOD licensed clinical psychologists," September 7, 1990; ACNP, 1991), a somewhat surprising stance for members of a group tasked with designing an ideal curriculum and one made more extraordinary by the fact that the ACNP was eventually awarded a $1.7 million contract to evaluate the outcome of the project. This award significantly increased the costs associated with the project, and costs became one of the reasons for its eventual demise.

Some controversy, however, was generated within the profession of psychology and reflects, then as now, that prescriptive authority is not a unanimously shared goal for the profession. Although most psychologists endorse the acquisition of prescriptive authority for the profession, approximately 25% of surveyed psychologists, over the course of a number of surveys conducted from the 1980s through the 1990s, have either disagreed or strongly disagreed with the notion that psychologists should be enabled to prescribe (representative surveys include those of Ax, Forbes, & Thompson, 1997; Bascue & Zlotowski, 1981; Cullen & Newman, 1997; Sammons, Gorny, Zinner, & Allen, 2000; Tatman, Peters, Greene, & Bongar, 1997) . Their opposition to prescriptive authority was vocal during the time of the PDP. The late Oakley Ray, a psychologist and the chair of the external evaluation panel appointed to oversee the PDP, was throughout the course of the project open in his dislike for it. In the same fashion, a small but active number of psychologists now campaign against state legislation to permit prescriptive authority for psychologists. This split between psychologists in support of and those opposed to prescriptive authority adds an interesting and perhaps unique element to the professional advocacy process. It is rare, and perhaps unheard of, that members of professions who advocate for an expanded scope of practice in state legislatures are opposed by members of their own profession. As stated, this dynamic was present from the inception of the PDP, and without question altered both its structure and interpretations of its success.

SHAPING OF THE CURRICULUM

In 1987, some members of the Congress, most notably Sen. Daniel K. Inouye (HI), who as a veteran severely injured in World War II has throughout his senatorial career taken a deep interest in the training of military health care providers, recommended that the DOD explore mechanisms to augment a shortage of skilled providers of psychotropic drugs by training psychologists to prescribe.[1] He was joined on the House side by Rep. John Murtha (PA) a retired U.S. Marine and an equally ardent advocate for military health care.

The language of that congressional mandate is instructive, insofar as it outlines the original intent of the legislation and provides a baseline to measure how the PDP was shaped by both political and professional forces. As described in Sammons and Brown (1997), the intent of the congressional language was to expand the utilization of nonphysician health care providers within DOD, specifically to

> . . . more aggressively utilize the clinical and administrative expertise of non-physician health care providers. The conferees further agree that the Department should expand the development of administratively separate psychology departments/services to include those treatment facilities in each of the Services providing psychology training programs. Given the importance of "battle fatigue," the conferees agree that the Department should establish a demonstration pilot training program under which military psychologists may be trained and authorized to issue appropriate psychotropic medications under certain circumstances. (U.S. House of Representatives, Report # 100-1002, p. 34, cited in Sammons & Brown, 1997, p. 107)

This congressional mandate was met with considerable opposition within military medicine, and 1 year later the Congress, noting the absence of progress in implementing the program, again directed the services to comply. This set in motion a series of events, the most important for our purposes is the convening of the Blue Ribbon Panel mentioned previously.

Arguments against the program were predictable. The reported shortage of military psychiatrists was argued not to actually exist, and it was held that there were more than ample psychiatrists to meet the mental health needs of service members. It was also argued that the training of psychologists did not adequately prepare them to be educated to use psychotropic drugs, the casuistry of which should be apparent to anyone involved in setting up a program to accomplish that very end. Within psychology, there was, at least in this author's impression, a relatively robust reluctance on the part of senior military psychologists to embrace a project that was different from other fellowship training models in military psychology, untried, and one that might

---

[1]Sen. Daniel K. Inouye was severely injured in the Italian campaign and suffered a traumatic amputation of his left arm. He spent many months under the care of military nurses and physicians, both during the war and during a lengthy rehabilitation period following. For his heroism in battle, he was later awarded the Congressional Medal of Honor.

threaten the rather fragile relationship between military psychologists and psychiatrists.[2]

However, a more interesting focus of opposition arose, and this centered on the absence of any historical antecedents for training psychologists to prescribe. It simply had not been done before, and Laskow and Grill (2003) rightly described this as a major impediment to the inception of the project. Those rare clinical psychologists who had prescribed, and there were several, such as Dr. Floyd Jennings who prescribed in the Indian Health Service in the 1980s, had all acquired their knowledge through on-the-job training and outside of any kind of formal program. Development of a curriculum was, then, relatively uncharted water and proved quickly to have numerous shoals. Should psychologists be trained according to the medical curriculum, or should they participate in educational models used in nursing or other health professions? Answers to these questions were not easily come by, but the first solution proposed within DOD was that psychologists could be trained to prescribe by using the curriculum for physician assistants (PAs). This curriculum possessed some inherent advantages, not the least of which was expedience. At 18 months the PA curriculum was relatively short. A well-developed military training program for PAs already existed at Ft. Sam Houston, Texas. This not only taught the fundamentals of allopathic medicine but also exposed trainees to the assessment and treatment of a variety of physical conditions—areas in which clinical psychologists admittedly had very little training.

Other models existed. The ACNP had published a model curriculum in psychopharmacology for psychiatric residents. Nurse practitioners also had models for advanced training in applied medicine. Allan Barclay of the Wright State School of Professional Psychology was contacted by the DOD and asked to devise a curriculum appropriate for psychologist prescribers. This curriculum involved a 2-month intensive didactic sequence of coursework in psychopharmacology and related subjects, followed by a 9-month proctored clinical experience interspersed with additional didactic material. Coursework was to be offered in a psychology-specific training program (held at Wright State) with proctored training in military psychiatric facilities. The Blue Ribbon Panel rejected the ACNP psychiatric residency curriculum on the grounds that it presumed extensive prior training as a physician and also because it had not been (and still has not been) completely implemented in any one training program. Nursing programs were rejected because they were not aimed at

---

[2]As in many health care delivery settings, military psychologists were on the whole relatively content to take a subordinate position to psychiatrists and other physicians. In the late 1980s, it was quite uncommon to have a psychologist serve as head of a military mental health department, psychiatrists almost exclusively filled this role.

training independently licensed providers. The PA model was considered, but it was also quickly rejected because it too did not aim to produce independent providers. A curriculum that came to be dubbed the "USUHS model," after the DOD's medical school, the Uniformed Services University of the Health Sciences, involving a 2-year sequence of coursework directly and indirectly related to psychopharmacology and a combined practical experience, was adopted in principle (unpublished minutes, Blue Ribbon Panel, "Training of military psychologists in limited psychopharmacology," February 27–28, 1990). The exact content of this curriculum remained unstated.

Although the Blue Ribbon Panel was meeting in the spring and summer of 1990, the Congress was exerting increasing pressure on DOD to implement a program. Consequently, in August of 1990, the first PDP fellows were enrolled in training. For expediency's sake it was decided to send two Army psychologists to Ft. Sam Houston in Texas to enroll in the PA curriculum, despite that this option had been rejected by the panel during its February meeting.

Several problems immediately emerged. First, exposing doctoral level, licensed providers to a curriculum then designed for individuals who were not routinely expected to possess a college education was problematic. Second, as discussed above, the program, although instilling excellent skills in practical prescribing, presumed that there would always be a degree of physician oversight over medication regimens—not a goal of the PDP. Finally, the program for PAs was almost exclusively focused on the treatment of physical illnesses. No specific training in mental disorders or their treatment existed, and no specific curriculum in psychopharmacology was a part of the PA curriculum. This would emerge as a problem in the adopted USUHS curriculum as well.

Recognition of the limits of the PA curriculum combined with disapproval of the panel and congressional pressure led to the abandonment of the PA approach. Within several months, the two fellows were recalled from Ft. Sam Houston to Walter Reed Army Medical Center (WRAMC), which had become the parent command for the program, and after this false start, a 9-month hiatus in training ensued.

Analysis of the Blue Ribbon Panel's deliberations will assist in laying to rest one persistent myth in regard to the PDP: that the participants were preselected on the basis of an extensive prior background in biological sciences. Indeed, the Blue Ribbon Panel was explicit in noting that participants with such backgrounds should be screened out so that the performance of those enrolled in the fellowship could be equated with that of psychologists in general. The panel also wrestled with the original congressional directive to focus on battle fatigue. It was widely acknowledged that battle fatigue—an imprecisely defined term that is the rough equivalent of combat stress or posttraumatic stress disorder—although being of keen interest to military mental health providers, was too limited an area on which to base a curriculum to prescribe. However, the psychiatry consultant to the Air Force Surgeon General advocated strict adherence to the 1988 authorization language and limiting training to only those psychotropic medications that would be used in the treatment of battle fatigue. This would obviously have limited training to a small armamentarium of agents and the subsequent utility of psychologists so trained, and this argument, likely made with the objective of decreasing the use of prescribing psychologists, did not prevail. The Blue Ribbon Panel, therefore, recommended that the goals of the training program be expanded to include a broader range of psychological disorders (unpublished minutes, Blue Ribbon Panel on the subject of training military psychologists in limited psychopharmacology, February 27–28, 1990).

This development was typical of how much of the training curriculum evolved in response to either political input or attempts to stop the program. An examination of the correspondence from the early days of the program shows the tensions that existed between those who were opposed to its inception on political grounds and those who, despite professional allegiances, sought to develop a robust and defensible curriculum. There was, for example, an early attempt to limit the practice of the graduates to active-duty military populations only. Because military populations tend to be younger, are in generally good psychological health, and are less likely to require psychotropic intervention, such a limitation would provide justification for an argument that the program was unnecessary. However, it soon became apparent to curriculum planners that no training program could be effectively designed that excluded other segments of the population and that this exclusion would result in ill-prepared trainees. Another early attempt sought to classify the demonstration project as clinical research, thereby requiring the enrollment of all patients treated by the participants in institutional review board–governed protocols with the likely result that such impediments to training would ensure abandonment of the project. All of these proposals were put forth by psychiatrists, who were essentially uniform in their opposition to the program and who controlled any military medical venue in which the participants would be trained.

The absence of training venues for prescribing psychologists was a major concern. Inpatient mental health units, more common in the late 1980s, were entirely the purview of psychiatry. Although all three branches of the service had, and continue to have, APA-approved predoctoral internships, these focused for the most part on outpatient care, with perhaps a single rotation on an inpatient mental health ward. As noted earlier, psychology departments were often located within psychiatry departments, and their leaders were generally subordinate to psychiatrists. This led to situations quite anomalous in the military, wherein a psychiatrist of junior rank would serve as the reporting officer for psychologists of much senior rank. Given the dominance of inpatient mental health by psychiatry, it is probable that the PDP trainees would have had a very difficult time finding appropriate training sites. However, in this instance, force majeure played a serendipitous role. In 1993, when the first fellows had completed their didactic training and scheduled to begin their full-time clinical experience, there was a significant shortage of psychiatric residents at WRAMC. Only four of a planned eight 2nd year residents entered the program that year. The necessity of staffing a large inpatient unit significantly lessened resistance to providing training slots for the participants, and the necessity of treating a full range of service members and their dependents, from adolescents to geriatrics, was largely responsible for the evaporation of the restriction to treat active duty members only.

In the summer of 1991 the first formal iteration of the PDP got underway, with an initial class of four fellows, two from the U.S. Army and two from the U.S. Navy. Time pressures and disagreement among curriculum planners meant that no courses specifically designed for psychopharmacology had been developed, although a panel consisting of members of the USUHS faculty met three times in spring 1991 to suggest appropriate alterations to the medical school curriculum. This panel was dominated by physicians, although two academic psychologists and two representatives from the Army's clinical psychology training program were represented (unpublished minutes; "Prescription Privileges for Clinical Psychologists Committee"; April 29, May 6, and May 23, 1991).

As might be expected, this group's focus was largely on that training model they were most familiar with—medical education. It is not surprising, then, that the

> consensus view emerged that a substantial course in Anatomy was indeed required, as well as Physiology, Biochemistry, Pharmacology, Neuro-anatomy, Pathology, Introduction to Clinical Medicine and Clinical Concepts. The physical exam and the taking of a medical history were deemed necessary. A small amount of additional material (beyond that required for the MD program) was thought to be necessary in certain areas of Clinical Pharmacology, such as legal aspects of prescription writing, and perhaps an extra session on the clinical pharmacology of psychotropic agents. (unpublished minutes, "Prescription Privileges for Clinical Psychologists Committee," May 6, 1991)

Although the absence of any more specific education in psychopharmacology beyond the "small amount of additional material" recommended might seem surprising today, it again must be reiterated that these planners were almost exclusively faculty and planners of a medical school. Limited by both time and by their pedagogical worldview, they fell back on what they knew—and trusted—best. In their last meeting, the panel attempted to address that the medical curriculum might not be best suited to meet the goals of the congressional mandate. They then proposed that in addition to the curriculum proposed above, that

> WRAMC develop a supplementary program (which could include USUHS components) of graduate level material drawn from the following areas:
> a. medical psychology
> b. behavioral pharmacology
> c. human genetics
> d. human context in health care
> e. introduction to immunology
> f. basic life support
> g. military applied physiology
> h. epidemiology and biometrics
> i. clinical pharmacology—a clinical experience stressing neuroactive drug use. (unpublished minutes, "Prescription Privileges for Clinical Psychologists Committee," May 23, 1991)

In other words, the committee, after proposing a model that comprised the vast majority of the standard medical curriculum, proceeded to expand this by recommending a supplementary program that essentially completed the remainder of medical education as then taught. That these planners were simply unable to move beyond the standard curriculum is amply reflected in their last recommendation—that clinical pharmacology education comprise a clinical experience that stressed neuroactive drug use—the first instance where any reference to psychopharmacology occurs in the entire proposed curriculum.

Thus, the first entrants into the PDP, instead of commencing a curriculum specifically designed to train psychologist prescribers, were enrolled in standard medical school courses with almost no modification, although they were exempt from certain portions of the entire medical curriculum. The influence of this model on future training of prescribing psychologists has been profound insofar that the basic presumption (that medical education was necessary to prescribe psychotropics) has been perpetuated in every model of clinical psychopharmacology for psychologists put forth since that time.

Once enrolled in medical school, it became immediately clear to the participants in the first cohort that the off-the-shelf medical school curriculum was not optimized to train psychologists to prescribe. Although the PDP fellows were excused from some of the coursework taken by 1st-year medical students (parasitology and medical zoology, epidemiology and biometrics, military studies and medical history; see Table 3.1), they took the fundamental courses of biochemistry, anatomy, and physiology in their entirety. That these fellows were not exposed to courses in pharmacology until the 2nd year of their curriculum should provide some index as to how inaptly suited the medical curriculum was to training psychologists to prescribe. Yet there was

TABLE 3.1
PDP Curriculum: Iteration 1, Year 1

Course	Contact hours
Courses taken by both PDP fellows and medical students[a]	
Anatomy I: Introduction to Cell and Tissue Biology, Embryology	
Anatomy II: Gross Anatomy of the Human Body	
Anatomy III: Anatomy of the Head, Neck, and Central Nervous System	
Anatomy IV: Microscopic Anatomy of Organs and Organ Systems	
Total for Anatomy I–IV	341
Biochemistry	160
Introduction to Clinical Medicine I	86
Medical Physiology	198
Total PDP	785
Courses taken only by medical students[b]	
Fundamentals of Diagnostic Parasitology, Medical Zoology	44
Epidemiology and Biometrics	66
Human Context in Health Care	66
Medical Psychology	44
Military Studies and Medical History	132
Military Medical Field Studies—Summer	110
Total	1,247

Note. USUHS = Uniformed Services University of the Health Sciences; PDP = Psychopharmacology Demonstration Project. From "The Department of Defense Psychopharmacology Demonstration Project: An evolving program for postdoctoral education in psychology" by M. T. Sammons & A. B. Brown, 1997, *Professional Psychology: Research and Practice, 28,* p. 110. Copyright 1997 by the American Psychological Association. [a]Hours include actual class and laboratory contact hours. [b]Hours are based on calculations from the USUHS catalog of approximately 22 contact hours per hour of course credit; may contain some nondirect contact hours.

extraordinary institutional resistance to modifying this curriculum to provide a more efficient vehicle for fellowship learning. The most telling example of such resistance came with opposition to the fellows' petition to be released from the Year 1 medical school course in medical psychology taught at USUHS. Although the fellows were eventually exempted from this requirement, the notion that doctorally trained, experienced clinical psychologists, all with extensive experience in health care service delivery should be required to take such a course demonstrated how reluctant planners were to alter the medical curriculum in any form.

The absence of a specific didactic sequence in psychopharmacology was a serious drawback to the fellowship. Not only did it mean that the courses psychologists took contained much material irrelevant to the prescription of psychotropics but it also reproduced a failing that persists in medical education to this day: that the didactic material specific to psychopharmacology in the standard medical curriculum is extraordinarily sparse and is limited to a few contact hours in a clinical pharmacology course.

Largely because of continued protests by the fellows enrolled in the program, successive modifications began to be incorporated into the curriculum

TABLE 3.2
PDP Curriculum: First Iteration, Year 2

Course	Contact hours
Courses taken by both PDF Fellows and medical students[a]	
Clinical Concepts	100
Clinical Pharmacology	47
Pathology	215
Pharmacology	86
Introduction to Clinical Medicine II	132
Total PDP	580
Courses taken only by medical students[b]	
Ethical, Legal, and Social Aspects of Medical Care	22
Human Behavior	88
Medical Microbiology and Infectious Diseases	220
Military Studies II	44
Preventive Medicine	66
Radiographic Interpretation	22
Total	462

Note. USUHS = Uniformed Services University of the Health Sciences; PDP = Psychopharmacology Demonstration Project. From "The Department of Defense Psychopharmacology Demonstration Project: An evolving program for postdoctoral education in psychology" by M. T. Sammons & A. B. Brown, 1997, *Professional Psychology, Research and Practice, 28,* p. 10. Copyright 1997 by the American Psychological Association. [a]Hours include actual class and laboratory contact hours. [b]Hours are based on calculations from the USUHS catalog of approximately 22 contact hours per hour of course credit; may contain some nondirect contact hours.

(see Table 3.2). In the third and final iteration of the curriculum, the off-the-shelf medical coursework had been reduced to a 1-year didactic sequence followed by a 1-year clinical experience. Extraneous courses had been deleted, other medical school course content had been modified to incorporate learning objectives of the PDP, and an additional course in clinical medicine and primary care was added. The total number of course hours diminished from 1,365 contact hours to 659.5 contact hours (Table 3.3). Clinical rotations were in inpatient, outpatient, and consultation-liaison services.

EXTERNAL SCRUTINY OF THE PDP

Opposition from organized medicine to the program had been intense. As early as 1991, competing language had been introduced in congressional appropriations bills to limit or stop the PDP. In addition to the ongoing monitoring provided by the ACNP, no fewer than three external groups were contracted to provide evaluations of the program and its goals. A report commissioned by the Office of the Undersecretary of Defense for Health Affairs was released in 1996 (Vector Research, 1996). This report concluded that the PDP was not only cost-effective but that it had achieved its goals of training safe and effec-

TABLE 3.3
PDP Final Curriculum

Course	Hours	Change from Iteration 2 (hours)
Anatomy	48	−6.0
Biochemistry	57	3.0
Neurosciences	54	12.0
Physiology	39	1.0
Pathophysiology	60	−42.0
Clinical Medicine	121	−3.5
Clinical Concepts	100	0.0
Pharmacology	83	0.0
Clinical Pharmacology	21	0.0
Psychopharmacology	21	0.0
Introduction to Primary Care	56	56.0
Total	660	19.5

Note. USUHS = Uniformed Services University of the Health Sciences; PDP = Psychopharmacology Demonstration Project. From "The Department of Defense Psychopharmacology Demonstration Project: An evolving program for postdoctoral education in psychology" by M. T. Sammons & A. B. Brown, 1997, *Professional Psychology, Research and Practice, 28*, p. 11. Copyright 1997 by the American Psychological Association.

tive psychologist prescribers. This report was immediately criticized by opponents to the project, and shortly thereafter, language was included in congressional appropriations bills to direct the U.S. Government Accountability Office (GAO; then called the U.S. General Accounting Office) to evaluate the cost effectiveness and necessity of the project. This report (GAO, 1997) was critical of the project. Although the auditors conceded that the program had successfully trained its participants, they focused on costs of the project. The assumptions behind their analysis were highly questionable. The GAO based their cost estimates on the estimated cost of training a medical student (a significant overestimation because the fellows took part of only portions of the medical school curriculum and did not engage in the expensive summer training given to military medical students) as well as nonincremental costs (e.g., the salaries of the fellows, ignoring that the fellows were simultaneously providing clinical services and filling critically short inpatient psychiatry resident positions). The GAO also failed to note that the single most expensive cost of the project was the contract, eventually totaling $1.7 million given to the ACNP to provide an external review of the project. The ACNP, an invited member–only organization representing the most renowned academics, researchers, and clinicians in psychopharmacology, were and remain without question the most expert group in this field. Academically they were the group most suited to developing and evaluating a curriculum in psychopharmacology. In selecting a panel to evaluate and guide the PDP, they, recognizing their inherent bias toward psychiatry, strove for balance by appointing an equal number of psychologists and psychiatrists with a psychologist as its head.

They provided thorough and reasonably nonjudgmental annual reports of the progress of the fellows and devised carefully thought-out written and clinical examinations to test their knowledge. Nevertheless, this group, like the earlier curriculum planning groups, was a medical group at heart and perpetuated the medical focus that remains central in training programs to this day.

As anticipated, the 1997 GAO report gave ammunition to the opponents of the project, whose criticism continued unflaggingly throughout the duration of the project. In 1996, congressional opponents successfully introduced congressional language denying further funding for the project, as they had attempted on at least two previous occasions. This time, this language survived conference committees and was included in the final legislation. At the end of the fourth training cycle, having produced 10 trained psychologist prescribers, the PDP ceased to exist.

The final evaluation of the ACNP, which had monitored, examined, and rated all enrolled fellows and which had remained central to discussions in regard to the structure of the training, was highly complimentary of the project.

> All 10 graduates of the PDP filled critical needs, and they performed with excellence wherever they were placed. It was striking to the Evaluation Panel how the graduates had filled different niches and brought unique perspectives to their various assignments. For example, a graduate at one site worked full time on an inpatient unit with his supervising psychiatrist. The psychiatrist said he preferred working with the graduate rather than with another psychiatrist because the prescribing psychologist contributed a behavioral, nonphysician, psychological perspective he got from no one else. On posts where there was a shortage of psychiatrists, the graduates tended to work side by side with psychiatrists, performing many of the same functions a "junior psychiatrist" might perform. In another location, a graduate was based in a psychology clinic but worked largely in a primary care clinic for dependents, thereby providing cost savings for care that otherwise would have been contracted out. Another graduate was the only prescriber for active duty sailors in a psychology clinic that was located near the ships at a naval base. Yet another graduate was to be transferred soon to an isolated base where he will be the only mental health provider. His medical backup will be primary care physicians. (ACNP, 1998, pp. 2–3)

Likewise, yet another GAO report, commissioned by the Congress (GAO, 1999), also spoke highly of the training afforded the participants and their activities on completion of the fellowship.

> The 10 PDP graduates seem to be well integrated at their assigned military treatment facilities. For example, the graduates generally serve in positions of authority, such as clinic or department chiefs. They also treat a variety of mental health patients; prescribe from comprehensive lists of drugs, or formularies; and carry patient caseloads comparable to those of

psychiatrists and psychologists at the same hospitals and clinics. Also, although several graduates experienced early difficulties being accepted by physicians and others at their assigned locations, the clinical supervisors, providers, and officials we spoke with at the graduates' current and prior locations—as well as a panel of mental health clinicians who evaluated each of the graduates—were complimentary about the quality of patient care provided by the graduates. (GAO, 1999, p. 2)

Nevertheless, the GAO continued to insist that the project was unneeded and the fellows did not contribute to overall readiness. The latter point is in certain respects supported. With only 10 graduates, the number of prescribing psychologists was too low to have an effect on overall shortages of mental health services. At the same time, several of the graduates were providing services in isolated environments where there were no psychiatric services available—thereby enhancing readiness at the local level.

THE PDP IN THE CONTEXT OF CURRENT INITIATIVES FOR PRESCRIPTIVE AUTHORITY

To this point, I have attempted to illustrate how the curriculum of the PDP was shaped and how politics and guild interests interfered with the development of an ideal training program best suited to train doctoral-level psychologists to prescribe. Many current opponents of prescriptive authority cite the PDP curriculum as a model or ideal curriculum, and they use it to make unfavorable comparisons to the prevailing curriculum based on recommendations from APA that forms the basis of most extant postdoctoral training programs. Some of these opponents have selectively abstracted certain language from the ACNP's final evaluation report that noted, "Virtually all graduates of the PDP considered the 'short-cut' programs proposed in various quarters to be ill-advised" (ACNP Final Report; American College of Neuropsychopharmacology, 1998, p. 3). It is important to understand in this context that the short-cut training programs we referred to were those proposing that psychologists could learn effective prescribing in curricula as short as 125 contact hours—approximately one quarter of the length of the APA-recommended curriculum, even before including the practical supervision component. All of the fellows were aware of the evolving APA curriculum that took shape during the mid-1990s through various task forces and work groups convened by the APA's Practice Directorate or APA's Board of Educational Affairs; indeed many of the graduates, including me, were consultants to such groups. What has been lost is the recognition that the PDP was devised, shaped, and evaluated by medicine, and it never became the specific training program in clinical psychopharmacology it was originally envisioned to be.

Cost

The issue of cost has remained quite lively in the decade since the PDP was ended. Opponents of prescriptive authority frequently detail in legislative testimony concerns in regard to the price of training the PDP fellows. Why an issue that was overblown at the time (given the unusual accounting methods of the GAO) should continue to be raised 11 years after the graduation of the last of the fellows is a bit mysterious. The most probable explanation is that finding little to criticize about the performance of the PDP graduates, opponents have again fallen back on a secondary argument that evades the central finding of all external evaluators—that psychologists can safely and effectively prescribe.

Unjustified Need for Psychologist Prescribers

One argument used against the PDP was that there was no shortage of appropriately trained psychiatrists in the military; therefore, the skills of prescribing psychologists were unnecessary. This argument has a curious history, for, even while the project was ongoing, military psychiatrists were arguing forcefully that their numbers were in critically short supply and that urgent recruitment efforts were required. A memo from the Psychiatry Consultant to the Air Force Surgeon General in 1996 was clear on this point, yet when the leadership of military psychiatry provided testimony to the GAO or other agencies contracted to evaluate the project, it was their repeated contention that there was an adequate supply of psychiatrists and other prescribers of psychotropics in the military environment. This detail is worth recalling because these arguments are repeatedly used today in front of state legislatures when organized psychiatry argues against the need for additional trained prescribers. These arguments have grown slightly more sophisticated in recent years. Although the supply of psychiatrists has not grown for many years it is now not common to hear that there are sufficient supplies of psychiatrists, but rather that appropriately trained primary care physicians can meet the demand, or that technologies, such as telehealth, can be leveraged by psychiatry to provide sufficient coverage of mental health needs. Both of these contentions are highly questionable. First, shortages of trained primary care physicians are commonly cited as a barrier to care for many Americans. Second, as noted earlier, the training of primary care physicians in psychopharmacology is generally quite limited. As has been repeatedly observed, the entire didactic curriculum for psychopharmacology training in basic medical education consists of 8 to 15 contact hours taken in the context of a broader pharmacology course. General physicians then get one 6-week clerkship on a psychiatry rotation, where hands-on patient training takes place. In practice, primary care physicians are unable to spend much time with patients, and the primary care model that presumes an initial visit with follow-up visits in intervals of months or more is generally not conducive to the treatment of most mental disorders. A recent study of visit length for patients with psychological disorders in a primary care found a mean visit length of 22.3 minutes (range 5.8–72 minutes; Geraghty, Franks, & Kravitz, 2007). The Geraghty et al. (2007) study is worth examining in some detail, as it provides an illustration of current practice patterns in primary care in standard outpatient (both health maintenance organization [HMO] and non-HMO) settings. These investigators examined the behavior of 152 primary care physicians who were exposed to two standardized patients, each of whom presented with depression, adjustment disorder, and a musculoskeletal complaint. Not unpredictably, patients of physicians with higher volume practice, those working in HMOs, and those who had more than 12 patients scheduled in a half-day clinic had visit lengths 15% to 27% shorter than the mean visit length of 22.3 minutes. Geraghty et al. found that the only variable that predicted the length of visit was whether the provider had a personal or vicarious experience with depression, in which case visit length was 11% longer. Of importance was the finding that a request for antidepressant medication did not increase the mean visit length, suggesting that when antidepressants were prescribed little time was spent advising the patient as to the use of such medication. Two rather extraordinary findings of this study were that out of a total of 294 encounters, inquiries about suicidal ideation were made in only 36% of visits and that length to follow-up visit was greater than 1 month in 55% of visits.

These data support the widely made observation that primary care physicians do not in general have sufficient time to deal with patients with psychological difficulties and that common elements of good practice with such patients (inquiries about suicidal ideation and regular follow-up) are not typical. They amplify many current arguments holding that in spite of the good intentions of primary care physicians, the structure of primary medical care does not permit appropriate diagnosis and management of common psychological disorders. The data provide support for the presence of specialty mental health providers in the primary care milieu, particularly those who have received training in the management of psychotropic agents.

PRESCRIBING IN TODAY'S MILITARY

Shortages of psychiatrists persist not only within civilian communities but also in the military. In part because of the wars in Iraq and Afghanistan, military mental health has been increasingly taxed to provide care to combatants and their families. Ongoing shortages in both military psychologists and psychiatrists have worsened as deployment-related stresses have caused many military medical providers to leave active duty. As might be expected, gaps in psychotropic medication management services continue to widen in the military and all three branches of the military have taken notice.

Credentialing

As of February 2009, the Army officially joined the ranks of the Navy and Air Force in outlining branch-specific policies and procedures for credentialing psychologists to prescribe psychotropic medications (Department of the Navy Bureau of Medicine and Surgery, 2003, p. 218; Secretary of the Air Force, 2007, p. 105; U.S. Army Medical Command, 2009). Although there are variations in the actual guidelines of the three branches, all three are consistent with the APA recommendations for prescribing (e.g., formal postdoctoral training, passing the Psychopharmacology Examination for Psychologists).

Although psychologists have been prescribing in the military since the first group of PDP graduates were successfully trained, until recently no formal guidelines were provided for non-PDP graduates in the military or civilian psychologists interested in prescribing in DOD medical centers and health clinics. In the past, credentialing was left up to the hospital commanders that provided oversight to the military treatment facility where the psychologist sought prescriptive privileges. Although the hospital commander is still the ultimate authority in credentialing matters, these new formal policies and procedures help facilitate the credentialing process for psychologists interested in prescribing and provides precedence and ammunition to counter those within the military health care community that are staunchly opposed to the allowing of prescriptive authority for psychologists.

Contributions in Deployed Settings

One significant contribution that prescribing psychologists make in the military is expanding the breadth and depth of psychopharmacotherapy provided in deployed settings (e.g., war zones such as Iraq, on ships). To date, all branches have deployed prescribing psychologists to Iraq in support of Operation Iraqi Freedom. Written and verbal reports by all of these psychologists have illustrated how they were able to provide a more comprehensive level of care as related to operating from a biopsychosocial model of treatment. In deployed settings, access to psychiatrists tends to be limited (e.g., remote bases in Iraq and Afghanistan) or nonexistent (e.g., naval ships). Prescribing psychologists are able to fill these gaps and effectively address the mental health concerns of service members, which maintains military readiness and contributes to the overall success of military operations.

Moore and McGrath (2007) provided a unique look at the challenges of providing adequate psychiatric care in Iraq, including excessive reliance on nonpsychiatric physicians and PAs for psychiatric services, the risks associated with transporting personnel to psychiatric services, and issues in continuity of care. They posited that increasing the number of military psychologists able to prescribe would improve the level and quality of care available for service members and potentially have a positive impact on prescriptive authority for psychologists at the state level.

Swords to Plowshares

A growing body of psychologists who have prescribed in the military will enter the civilian psychological community as seasoned prescribers. These psychologists will bring a proven track record of safe and effective prescribing to the civilian sector. This provides strength for the prescriptive authority movement at the state level. They will also bring experience, knowledge, and respect to the legislative process. Military prescribing psychologists will make highly reputable and competent advocates and powerful influences in developing and securing state prescribing laws.

It is thus clear that the principal aim of the PDP—expanding the availability of skilled military prescribing psychologists—was legitimate at the inception of the project and paved the way for prescribing psychologists in the military as well as the civilian sector.

CONCLUSION

Despite the passage of time, the PDP remains a touchstone in current arguments in regard to prescriptive authority. Insofar as well over 500 psychologists have been subsequently trained in psychology-specific curricula that adhere to current standards as proposed by the APA, it is a bit curious that so much focus continues on a program that trained only 10 psychologists. Being the first organized training program no doubt accounts for much of this, as does the fact that it was a military training program and thus inherently in the public eye and prone to controversy (readers in 2010 have no need to be reminded of the highly controversial nature of some components of military mental health). However, perhaps more important was that it has been the only program for which unequivocal documentation of success exists. Subsequent training programs have not been subject to the same degree of external scrutiny. This is unfortunate, for these programs more closely resemble ideal education in clinical psychopharmacology for psychologists in that they address the issue of psychotropic use from a model that is fundamentally rooted in psychological, not medical, science.

Ultimately, success is not measured by reports of external consultants. Our clearest index of success is that there are now over 100 psychologist prescribers in Louisiana, New Mexico, and the federal sector who have an accumulating track record of safe and effective prescribing. The fundamental medical argument that patient safety would be imperiled by psychologist prescribers has not been proven to be true. Prescribing psychologists are now routinely credentialed in all three branches of the armed services, and they are trained in fellowship programs both within and outside of the DOD. The struggle for success in state legislatures continues, but if rationality and a recognition of the unmet needs of the public prevail over narrow guild interests, further expansion of training of psychologists in this important endeavor is inevitable.

REFERENCES

American College of Neuropsychopharmacology. (1991). Prescribing privileges for non-physicians in the military: Accepted as a consensus statement by the ACNP council, March 22, 1991. *Neuropsychopharmacology, 4*, 290–291.

American College of Neuropsychopharmacology. (1998). *DoD prescribing psychologists: External analysis, monitoring, and evaluation of the program and its participants*. Nashville, TN: Author.

Ax, R. K., Forbes, M. R., & Thompson, D. D. (1997). Prescription privileges for psychologists: A survey of predoctoral interns and directors of training. *Professional Psychology, Research and Practice, 28*, 509–514. doi:10.1037/0735-7028.28.6.509

Bascue, L. O., & Zlotowski, M. (1981). Psychologists' attitudes about prescribing medications. *Psychological Reports, 48*, 645–646.

Cullen, E. A., & Newman, R. (1997). In pursuit of prescription privileges. *Professional Psychology, Research and Practice, 28*, 101–106. doi:10.1037/0735-7028.28.2.101

DeLeon, P. H., Folen, R. A., Jennings, F. L., Willis, D. J., & Wright, R. H. (1991). The case for prescription privileges: A logical evolution of professional practice. *Journal of Clinical Child Psychology, 20*, 254–267. doi:10.1207/s15374424jccp2003_4

DeLeon, P. H., Fox, R. E., & Graham, S. R. (1991). Prescription privileges: Psychology's next frontier? *American Psychologist, 46*, 384–393. doi:10.1037/0003-066X.46.4.384

DeLeon, P. H., Sammons, M. T., & Sexton, J. L. (1995). Focusing on society's real needs: Responsibility and prescription privileges? *American Psychologist, 50*, 1022–1032. doi:10.1037/0003-066X.50.12.1022

Department of the Navy Bureau of Medicine and Surgery. (2003). *Credentials review and privileging program (BUMED Instruction 6320.66D)*. Washington, DC: Author.

Dunivin, D. L., & Orabona, E. (1999). Department of Defense Psychopharmacology Demonstration Project: Fellows' perspectives on didactic curriculum. *Professional Psychology, Research and Practice, 30*, 510–518. doi:10.1037/0735-7028.30.5.510

Geraghty, E. M., Franks, P., & Kravitz, R. L. (2007). Primary care visit length, quality, and satisfaction for standardized patients with depression. *Journal of General Internal Medicine, 22*, 1641–1647. doi:10.1007/s11606-007-0371-5

Laskow, G. B., & Grill, D. J. (2003). The Department of Defense Experiment: The Psychopharmacology Demonstration Project. In M. T. Sammons, R. U. Paige, & R. F. Levant (Eds.), *Prescriptive authority for psychologists: A history and guide* (pp. 77–101). Washington, DC: American Psychological Association. doi:10.1037/10484-005

Moore, B., & McGrath, R. (2007). How prescriptive authority for psychologists would help service members in Iraq. *Professional Psychology, Research and Practice, 38*, 191–195. doi:10.1037/0735-7028.38.2.191

Newman, R., Phelps, R., Sammons, M. T., Dunivin, D. L., & Cullen, E. A. (2000). Evaluation of the Psychopharmacology Demonstration Project: A retrospective analysis. *Professional Psychology, Research and Practice, 31*, 598–603. doi:10.1037/0735-7028.31.6.598

Sammons, M. T., & Brown, A. B. (1997). The Department of Defense Psychopharmacology Demonstration Project: An evolving program for postdoctoral education in psychology. *Professional Psychology, Research and Practice, 28*, 107–112. doi:10.1037/0735-7028.28.2.107

Sammons, M. T., Gorny, S. W., Zinner, E. S., & Allen, R. P. (2000). Prescriptive authority for psychologists: A consensus of support. *Professional Psychology, Research and Practice, 31*, 604–609. doi:10.1037/0735-7028.31.6.604

Sammons, M. T., Sexton, J. L., & Meredith, J. (1996). Basic science training in psychopharmacology: How much is enough? *American Psychologist, 51*, 230–234. doi:10.1037/0003-066X.51.3.230

Secretary of the Air Force. (2007). *Medical quality operations* (Air Force Instruction 44-119). Washington, DC: Author.

Tatman, S. M., Peters, D. B., Greene, A. L., & Bongar, B. (1997). Graduate students' attitudes toward prescription privileges training. *Professional Psychology, Research and Practice, 28*, 515–517. doi:10.1037/0735-7028.28.6.515

Thomas, C. R., & Holzer, C. E. (2006). The continuing shortage of child and adolescent psychiatrists. *Journal of the American Academy of Child and Adolescent Psychiatry, 45*, 1023–1031. doi:10.1097/01.chi.0000225353.16831.5d

U.S. Army Medical Command. (2009, February 13). *Policy and procedures for credentialing and privileging clinical psychologists to prescribe medications*. Fort Sam Houston, TX: Author.

U.S. Government Accountability Office. (1997). *Defense health care: Need for more prescribing psychologists is not adequately justified* (GAO/HEHS-97-83). Washington, DC: Author.

U.S. Government Accountability Office. (1999). *Prescribing psychologists: DOD demonstration participants perform well but have little effect on readiness or costs* (GAO-HEHS-99-98). Washington, DC: Author.

Vector Research. (1996). *Cost-effectiveness and feasibility of the DOD Psychopharmacology Demonstration Project. Final report*. Arlington, VA: Author.

II

GENERAL PRACTICE ISSUES

4

NUTS AND BOLTS OF PRESCRIPTIVE PRACTICE

GLENN A. ALLY

After you complete your postdoctoral training in clinical psychopharmacology, pass the Psychopharmacology Examination for Psychologists (PEP), and possibly spend a year completing a supervised clinical experience in pharmacotherapy, you are ready to begin prescribing. So, what happens next? Of course, a great deal of the answer depends on the statutes, rules, and regulations of the body that will authorize you to prescribe. The U.S. military has different rules and regulations in regard to prescribing than do the states. There are psychologists prescribing within the Indian Health Service (IHS), where the rules and regulations can differ not only from state standards but even between the various service units of IHS. These standards may govern a variety of aspects of prescribing: under what conditions, with what populations, in what facilities or settings, and with what formulary. As a psychologist with prescriptive authority about to embark on writing prescriptions, it should go without saying that it is extremely important to familiarize yourself with the rules and regulations of the governing body that authorizes prescriptive authority in your state and setting.

In this chapter, I explore some simple and practical techniques, procedures, or both, that may make using this new skill a little easier for you and perhaps for even your office staff. Some may be more relevant than others to you, but most will be helpful to some extent. The recommendations and tips in this chapter are, by no means, the only way to go about prescribing. They are based on my experience as a prescribing psychologist and countless hours of discussion with other colleagues who have chosen to take up the practice of pharmacotherapy.

A NEW IDENTITY

It may seem like a trivial issue, but new prescribers must reconsider their professional identity, or at least how they present themselves to the public and other health care professionals. In addition, your state psychology licensing board may want some means of differentiating those psychologists with prescriptive authority from those who do not prescribe. This can be accomplished in a number of ways. State psychology licensing boards may issue separate numbers with the certificate of prescriptive authority or perhaps decide to include identifying letters after existing license numbers.

Military psychologists with prescriptive authority trained through the Department of Defense Psychology Demonstration Project (PDP) are called *prescribing psychologists*. At the time of the development of the PDP, the military chose the title to be used, and the psychologists involved in that training had little input into the nomenclature. For some, the issue of what to be called will be settled by the statute passed in your respective state. At the present time, two states have prescriptive authority statutes and identify such psychologists by different terms. In New Mexico, psychologists with prescriptive authority are called prescribing psychologists. In Louisiana, which currently has the largest number of psychologists with prescriptive authority, they are called *medical psychologists*.

With regard to Louisiana, several different titles were considered. Psychologists with prescriptive authority believed the term *medical psychologist* more accurately reflected the level of training and expertise possessed by those individuals. Proponents of the designation *medical psychologist* believed *prescribing psychologist* described a behavior and did not reflect the scope of what psychologists with prescriptive authority actually do. There were those who were hesitant and fearful that the medical community would oppose this nomenclature and that legislation with the term *medical psychologist* as a professional descriptor would not pass. However, most agreed that the medical establishment and psychiatry in particular would oppose any bill regardless of what term was used.

The choice was a relatively simple one for Louisiana psychologists who were pursuing prescriptive authority. However, the issue was, and is today, not without controversy within our profession as a whole. For example, some health psychologists have used the term *medical psychology* when practicing in medical settings (e.g., hospitals, clinics, medical schools). However, *medical* is part of what psychologists with prescriptive authority actually do, not the setting in which they work. Medical psychologists in Louisiana not only prescribe, but they also order laboratory work and diagnostic studies such as computed tomography scans, magnetic resonance imaging studies, electrocardiograms, and so forth. They do limited physical examinations and monitor and adjust treatment plans according to patients' physical and psychological responses to medications. They must also be proficient in responding to medication-induced side effects, monitoring physical diseases, and suggesting physical interventions when deemed appropriate.

Regardless of the terms used to describe psychologists with prescriptive authority, what must be remembered is that now, with this authority, come the responsibility and the liability for decisions in regard to certain aspects of patients' medical and psychological well-being. Knowing what to call oneself will help those in the public and professionals in the health care setting to identify those psychologists with this very special expertise.

A FEW HURDLES TO CLEAR

Preparing to write that first prescription is an exciting moment. Unfortunately, there are a few hurdles to jump beforehand. First, make some inquiries of colleagues who have already received prescriptive authority in the state or federal agency where you intend to prescribe. It is very important to determine what licenses or certificates you may need in addition to your certificate of prescriptive authority.[1] You will also need to know about the renewal period for each.

Once you have obtained the required state or local approval, the next step in the process is to apply for the Controlled Substance Registration Certificate from the U.S. Department of Justice Drug Enforcement Administration, or DEA number. James Quillin, who is a former president of the Louisiana Academy of Medical Psychologists (LAMP), worked with the Louisiana branch of the DEA so they would recognize medical psychologists as a prescribing profession. In DEA nomenclature, medical psychologists are currently considered *midlevel practitioners,* a class that includes all prescribing professions except medicine, dentistry, veterinary, and podiatry; as such, the

---

[1]For example, a Louisiana Controlled and Dangerous Substance License is required for anyone who manufactures, distributes, dispenses, prescribes, and/or conducts research with pharmaceuticals in Louisiana. The license is issued by the Louisiana Board of Pharmacy and verifies the licensee's agreement to allow inspection of the premises and full compliance with the rules and regulations of the Uniform Controlled Substances Law.

class includes a number of professions such as nursing that prescribe at less than the doctoral level. It would be desirable if in the future medical psychologists were elevated to the level of four practitioner professions.

The application process is relatively straightforward and can be accomplished online at http://www.deadiversion.usdoj.gov. In the process of filling out the application for the DEA registration number, you will be asked to supply any state certificate or license numbers that may be required in your state. This is why it is recommended you get all state certificates or licenses first.

The DEA number is to be supplied to pharmacies when writing, telephoning in, or electronically providing prescriptions for your patients. It is necessary when prescribing controlled substances, and many agencies will require that you supply your DEA number during their credentialing process.

This may sound trivial, but you will need something on which to write your prescriptions. Check state statutes for what constitutes a valid prescription. Additionally, different agencies may have different requirements. For example, Medicaid in Louisiana requires prescriptions to be written on paper that, much like paper currency, is very difficult to duplicate. That same requirement does not apply to prescriptions written for individuals with other types of coverage. Consequently, you want to comply with the most rigorous relevant requirements when ordering prescription pads. With regard to size, shape, color, and style, there are a variety of prescription pads available through medical supply companies. In the past, some pharmaceutical companies supplied prescription pads free of charge to prescribers. Given the recent concerns over gifts from the pharmaceutical industry, this may no longer occur, but prescription pads ordered from medical supply catalogs are relatively inexpensive. Some prescribers have their DEA number preprinted on the prescription pads, although you can write it in.

Last, make sure you have professional liability insurance that covers your actions as a prescriber. At this time, there is only one insurance company writing professional liability coverage for psychologists with prescriptive authority. LAMP turned to the American Psychological Association Insurance Trust (APAIT) for assistance with this important issue. LAMP began negotiations to determine what would be an appropriate rate for professional liability insurance for psychologists with prescriptive authority. It is obvious that there were no data in regard to psychologists who were prescribing in the civilian sector on which to base a rate. In the end a premium increase of 15% was negotiated for psychologists with prescriptive authority. It is important to understand that this increase only applies to psychologists with prescriptive authority. Though opponents of prescriptive authority in our own profession often complain that liability rates for all psychologists will increase as a result, that claim is simply untrue.

At the present time, you must belong to APA to apply for liability insurance through APAIT. Until you obtain professional liability coverage for your activities as a prescriber, it is wise to refrain from prescribing or ordering medications for your patients. It is also important to remember that at this time the risk pool for prescribing psychologists is quite small. As a result, any claim could substantially increase costs. It is important that all psychologists prescribing outside the military recognize that any lapses in professional judgment could have profound economic implications for all prescribers until the number of psychologists with prescriptive authority is substantially larger than it is now.

CLINICAL AND BUSINESS PRACTICE ISSUES

Now that you are ready to start prescribing, there a few clinical and business practice issues you should consider. First, what do you need to revise on the intake form that you have been using all these years? For psychologists with prescriptive authority, the intake evaluation needs to include many more items in regard to medical history, vital signs, a more detailed accounting of current medications and medication allergies, and other health information. Even aspects of medical history you have always gathered need to be addressed in new ways. For example, you have probably always asked about pregnancy history and children. As a medical or prescribing psychologist, you will also want to know whether the patient is breastfeeding, as all psychotropics are found in breast milk to varying degrees. Other important information to consider is the last time a patient had a medical examination, laboratory work, or other relevant medical testing. In light of the additional intake information needed as well as additional paperwork, you might consider extending your first appointment with each new patient. Some clinicians provide their intake evaluation paperwork online so that the prospective patient can download the intake form, fill it out at home, and bring it with them to the appointment.

You may want to obtain some medical information in your office, such as the patient's vital signs and weight. This medical information may not be necessary for those patients who do not receive prescriptions; therefore, some decisions must be made about whether this information will be obtained on all patients or only those for whom you intend to prescribe medications. That can be hard to decide before seeing the patient, so again, plan for this possibility.

It may be desirable to differentiate in your medical records between those patients for whom you are and are not prescribing medications. Some simple procedures can assist with this task, such as different colored file folders for the two groups. However, it is often difficult to know before seeing the patient whether or not you will prescribe, and in many offices and clinics the file basics are compiled prior to seeing the patient. Another possibility is using different colored stickers on the folder, for example, placing a red sticker on the charts of those patients for whom you have written prescriptions. Such stickers can be used for other discriminations as well. For example, one color sticker can be used for patients receiving psychotherapy alone, another color for psychological evaluations, and yet another color for those patients for whom you are prescribing. It will also be important to have some way to identify those patients that have a medication or food allergy.

Other forms and means of documentation will become necessary when adding prescriptive authority to your practice. Laboratory forms and reports, vital sign graphs, metabolic base rates, and other pieces of information will have to be incorporated into your patients' charts. When using antipsychotics, a periodic assessment of extrapyramidal symptoms (e.g., involuntary movements, tremors and rigidity, restlessness) is advisable. Consequently, using a measure such as the Abnormal Involuntary Movement Scale (AIMS; Munetz & Benjamin, 1988) periodically can be beneficial. This instrument is available in various forms online. It will also be necessary to periodically order and assess blood serum levels for certain pharmacological agents. You will also need enough equipment to do a limited physical examination. You may find the following helpful: pen light, reflex hammer, stethoscope, sphygmomanometer, thermometer, and scale.

Another practice issue to address is how to deal with the samples provided to you by drug representatives. If you are going to keep samples in your office, check with your state guidelines for proper storage of these substances. For example, controlled substances will likely need to be stored in a locked cabinet or safe. If you are not sure where to find this information, check with the board of pharmacy in your state. They may have the relevant information or at least be able to tell you where it might be found. In addition, you should go through the sample cabinet periodically to ensure that the samples have not expired.

SELECTING THE RIGHT PATIENT

I know we all want that first patient to whom we prescribe to be just the most perfect patient with some very difficult mental health issue; we make the absolutely spot-on diagnosis; develop a terrific treatment plan that involves the use of psychotropic medication; we write the perfect prescription; the patient takes the medication exactly as we prescribed it; and 2 weeks later the patient returns just to tell us that he or she is "cured." I guess you know it seldom works out that way.

Selecting the right patient for the use of medication intervention sounds like it is a simple thing to do. Perhaps for physicians and other prescribers it may present as a simple choice because the use of medication is either the only or the major tool available to them, and their experiences during internship and residency have made them comfortable with the whole idea of prescribing. We have not had the same experiences and opportunities as our physician colleagues. Additionally, the decision making may be a little more complex for medical and prescribing psychologists.

Psychologists are fortunate to have a variety of tools to address the issues of mental illness. Psychologists are more apt to recognize what may be the right tool even when that psychologist is not personally proficient in a specific therapeutic technique. For example, a psychologist may recognize when a psychodynamic approach might be optimal even if he or she has not maintained their expertise to use such an approach in an individual therapy setting. In such instances it is imperative to recognize that referral to a professional proficient in this approach would be proper. This makes decision making for medical and prescribing psychologists potentially a little more complex. Therefore, deciding whether to prescribe for that patient may not be as easy as it sounds.

Then there are patient characteristics that may enter into your decision making to write that first prescription. Obviously, one of the more important patient considerations is whether this particular patient will benefit from the addition of psychotropic medication. If you feel the patient will indeed benefit, then other considerations are also important.

One such factor that bears on the decision to prescribe is patient expectations. Often when patients know that a professional prescribes medications they expect that they will leave that professional's office with prescriptions. Research indicates that a sizeable minority of patients ask for drugs by brand name (Peck et al., 2004). Typically, such drugs tend to be newer, more expensive ones for which safety information may be incomplete because they are early in their life cycles. According to Peck et al. (2004), not only are consumers asking for medications by name but substantial numbers are also receiving them. Patients who did not receive the desired medications even reported lower satisfaction with the interaction, and up to one third of them indicated that they would switch doctors if they did not receive the medication they requested.

It is important to recognize that some of these patient expectations and characteristics can influence issues such as compliance, development of side effects, and efficacy. Astute clinicians will spend time in the session discussing specific medications, and even after deciding on a medication will discuss patient expectations with regard to the use of medications in general. Some patients have preconceived notions, good and bad, about medications based on information from television advertising and other sources. You should be alert to the advertising by pharmaceutical companies for certain medications. You should also pay attention to other sources, such as some of the advertising done by plaintiffs' attorneys seeking to have patients become part of class action suits involving certain medications.

Other factors that might influence selecting that right first patient include referral sources and settings. Inevitably, once you begin prescribing, some of your physician colleagues will see this as an opportunity to refer some of the "problem patients" whom they have unsuccessfully attempted to treat. Many of these patients will come to your office already on psychotropic medications prescribed by their primary care physicians. In such cases, they may need medications adjusted rather than new prescriptions.

Likewise, in hospital settings, patients will often move from one service to another. For example, some geriatric patients need orthopedic surgery after they have fallen and sustained a hip fracture. They will initially be on the orthopedic unit for immediate recovery from the surgical intervention. Geriatric patients often experience difficulty sleeping in such unfamiliar surroundings and are prescribed something for sleep. With the longer recovery, decreased mobility, and temporary loss of independence, it is not uncommon for there to be some depression observed. After an appropriate recovery time on the orthopedic service, patients may be transferred to the physical medicine and rehabilitation service. By this time, patients may be on medications for insomnia, depression, anxiety, diminished appetite, and other symptoms. If you are in a hospital setting, you may find yourself adjusting or consolidating medications in situations such as this.

PREPARING THE PATIENT FOR USE OF MEDICATION

Once you find that perfect first patient to which you will prescribe medications, the next step is to get that patient ready. He or she should be informed of the risks and benefits of the medications you are considering. If the patient is taking other medications, certainly you will want to discuss any potential interactions. You can provide this information verbally, present prepared information from other sources, or use a combination of both. In addition to discussing risks and benefits and potential interactions, it is also important to inform patients of potential interactions with substances not normally considered, such as tobacco, alcohol, and over-the-counter products, and herbal treatments. The patient should also be informed if the medication chosen can produce sedation. If sedating medications are prescribed, obviously the patient should be warned about driving or operating high-speed, hazardous equipment. Document in the patient's record that you informed him or her of the risk.

In preparing patients for the use of psychotropic medication, it is important to communicate that medication may not be the sole answer to their presenting problems. In conveying this message, use examples that patients are able to understand. For example, you can use the analogy of patients with diabetes, for whom taking insulin is not enough but must be accompanied by changes in their diet. So, too, patients taking psychotropic medications may also need to monitor thinking patterns, exercise, and attend therapy sessions regularly. The most salient point to communicate is that medication helps to create the setting in which patients can either use their existing skills to deal with problems or can learn new skills.

DISCUSSING SIDE EFFECTS

As some readers may recall, physicians in years past were somewhat reluctant to discuss potential side effects of medications with patients. They had little difficulty discussing some of the potentially serious side effects, but the milder side effects were seldom mentioned. The thinking was that by discussing potential side effects the power of suggestion would increase the risk. That has changed in an age of informed consent.

Of course, as a psychologist you already know that discussing the risks and benefits of the intervention that you are recommending is extremely important for patients to be able to provide informed consent. There are a variety of software programs that can assist with this process by providing printouts in regard to the medication that you and your patient choose. Proper discussion and education can reduce patients' fears and concerns about medications and can enhance a sense of empowerment and responsibility.

KEEPING TRACK OF PRESCRIPTIONS

As with any other aspect of the diagnostic decision-making and treatment planning process, offering medication as a treatment should be recorded in the patient's record in some manner. There may be state statutes or regulations defining the documentation that is required in patient charting of medications and prescriptions. Make sure to familiarize yourself with the requirements. Bear in mind that requirements that govern prescribing may be found in regulations that govern the practice of medicine or pharmacy rather than psychology. You might ask a physician colleague to direct you to the relevant information.

There are various ways to document this information. You can make and keep a copy of the prescription in the chart and even have the patient sign the copy. A copy is particularly useful if you are concerned that the patient may alter the prescription. Some prescription pads produce carbon duplicates of prescriptions. Keep in mind that you will have to document both the prescriptions that you write and the prescriptions and refills that you call in to pharmacies.

If changes are made to medications during an inpatient hospitalization, it is important to document this in both the medication order section of the chart and in the progress notes. Also add an order for the nurse to fax a copy of the progress note to your office. In that way you will know whom you saw in the hospital the prior evening, what you did, and any medication changes you may have made.

Finally, you will in all likelihood receive phone calls in regard to medications and refills when your office is closed and when you are on call. Writing a short note in regard to the phone call is extremely helpful. You may want to invest in a personal digital assistant for this chore as random slips of paper can easily get lost. Once you return to the office, make a note of these transactions in the appropriate charts.

You will find the method that works best for you and your practice. The important message here is that regardless of the setting in which you may practice, there is no substitute for good documentation. This is especially true when it comes to documenting the prescribing of medications as part of everyday practice.

MONITORING PROGRESS

As a medical or prescribing psychologist, you will find that patients vary in terms of the amount of monitoring they require. Of course, this is not unique to being a prescriber, but the monitoring process is a little different because there is additional information involved.

Do not be afraid to ask questions of patients who are taking medications. When patients have difficulty with the medication, they will generally not hesitate to let you know what problems they may be experiencing. In fact, they may ask whether the new symptom they are experiencing could be a side effect of the medication. Even so, it is always important that you ask questions. These problems may be signs of another medical problem for which referral would be appropriate. Keep in mind that patients do not always report symptoms in the way the textbooks and package inserts describe. For example, one patient may report she is doing fine with her sertraline but then indicate she has been experiencing headaches lately. On further questioning, the patient notes that she usually experiences these headaches on awakening. Some selective serotonin reuptake inhibitors have been associated with a rare side effect of bruxism (i.e., an involuntary habit of clenching or grinding the teeth typically during sleep), and a different medication may alleviate the headaches. The point is that in addition to asking questions about typical side effects, it is important to ask generally about health. It is also important to ask not only whether the medication has been helpful but also how it has been helpful.

Various tools have been suggested for monitoring progress quantitatively, and these tools can contribute to risk management. Hatfield and Ogles (2004) provided information about the most commonly used outcome measures. More recently, the Patient-Reported Outcomes Measurement Information System (PROMIS; Castel et al., 2008) has been suggested as a general tool for evaluating progress in treatment.

If patients are being titrated to a higher dose of medication, you should review potential side effects. You should also regularly review the process of weaning medications rather than having the patient discontinue a medication abruptly. This can be particularly important when a patient feels better or when the patient is dissatisfied with the effect and may decide to discontinue the medication unilaterally.

COMPLIANCE CONCERNS

Suppose you are writing prescriptions and you realize the patient for whom you prescribed paroxetine 40 mg daily has decided that if a little is good, more would be a whole lot better. The patient has decided to take two instead of one. This brings up the issue of compliance or adherence. There is a large literature that explores factors related to compliance, and it is a very good idea to become familiar with some of this literature. For example, in a British study of compliance, Cooper et al. (2007) found that 34.2% of patients taking psychotropic medications reported incomplete adherence to their psychiatric medications. Of those who were noncompliant, 37.4% reported forgetting, losing their medications, or running out of their medications. Another 24.6% thought that their medications were unnecessary. Another 18.9% reported a reluctance to take drugs, and 14.2% were noncompliant because of side effects. Other studies reported much higher rates of adherence problems because of side effects (e.g., Ashton, Jamerson, Weinstein, & Wagoner, 2005).

Many issues influence compliance, not the least of which is patient characteristics. There are obvious reasons for noncompliance, such as the patient forgetting to take the drug or how to take the drug. Patients may deny they have the disorder or problem with which they have been diagnosed, or they may believe that the drug cannot help. Some patients may have difficulty paying for the medications prescribed. Others are experiencing drug interactions, side effects, or both but do not discuss these with their prescribing professional. Some patients are cognitively impaired and unable to follow instructions. Still another factor is a chronic condition that varies in intensity for which patients believe they should vary the amount of medication taken.

Personality characteristics can influence compliance. For example, patients with paranoid features may be suspicious about their medications, your motives for prescribing them, or both. Patients with borderline personality disorder may stop medications abruptly if they experience even minimal to mild side effects. Those with obsessive–compulsive features may become so vigilant for potential side effects that they find it difficult to relax. Each of these patients may require a different form of education and reassurance regarding side effects and compliance.

As you know, the patient may not experience maximum benefit from some psychotropic medications immediately. Maximum benefits may actually be experienced days or weeks later, although side effects may occur much earlier. Patients can become noncompliant with medications or abandon the pharmacotherapy prematurely if they experience even mildly bothersome side effects. Such patients may be more likely to continue adherence if they are properly educated and prepared for some of the potential problems. Side effects may occur throughout the course of use of some medications. Thus, the process of monitoring, education, and discussion in regard to psychotropic medication should be an ongoing one.

Regardless of the reason for noncompliance, you should have discussions with your patients about the potential problems of not taking medications as they are prescribed and educate them throughout the course of treatment. Having frequent discussions about their medications will help to reduce noncompliance.

MANAGING THE DRUG SEEKER

With the "good" sometimes comes some "bad." Inevitably that bad will find their way to your office, in the form of the drug seeker. You probably already know such a patient, but now you may be responsible for that patient's psychotropic medication. It has been difficult to agree on a definition of drug seeking. It seems to be one of those things that is difficult to define, but you know it when you see it. It generally involves patients' manipulative, demanding behaviors to obtain certain medications. Drug seekers often know the medication they want and present themselves so that the only possible solution to their presenting problem is prescription of a controlled substance.

Here is a partial list of some of the more creative arguments I have heard:

- I had a hole in my pocket and lost my medication bottle.
- My dog ate my medication (as you hear the dog barking in the background).
- My son was playing with my bottle of medication, and I can't find it (Scary!).
- My mother was holding my medications, and she has Alzheimer's.
- My wife and I got into a fight, and she flushed my medicine down the toilet.
- I lost my order for refills during Hurricane Katrina (5 years ago).
- I left my medication on the plane.

Granted, some excuses are going to be valid, and it can be difficult to determine who is truthful and who is not. Here are a few situations that should raise red flags for you:

- claiming to have a high tolerance to drugs;
- calling in frequently for refills;
- visiting the emergency room frequently;
- claiming to lose prescriptions;
- running out of medications too early;
- using the prescription of others or "borrowing" medications;
- shopping for doctors;
- having prescriptions from multiple prescribers;
- discounting nonpreferred drugs or treatments; and
- splitting doctors.

Drug-seeking patients are quite adept at using whatever technique works with a particular prescriber. If a prescriber capitulates when the patient cries, the patient will learn to use tears to manipulate. If the prescriber relents after a display of anger, then that becomes the drug seeker's "ace in the hole." Drug seekers are quite good at manipulation, and many prescribers are good at being manipulated. Are there some things that you can do as a prescriber to try to minimize the opportunity for abuse of your prescriptions? It turns out the answer is *yes*. Remember to have a clear indication for the medication being contemplated as an intervention. Doing an early risk assessment, regularly monitoring for compliance, documenting properly, and intervening when indicated can minimize the potential for abuse. Additionally, limiting the use of benzodiazepines and recognizing the utility of behavioral interventions at the outset may set the stage for minimizing the abuse potential. You are, after all, a psychologist and have alternative interventions that may be extremely helpful as well.

If you have any suspicion that there is high potential for abuse, ask the patient to agree to certain things:

1. only one prescriber for the patient's psychotropic medications;
2. only one pharmacy for filling medications;
3. no changing of dosages without discussing the change first;
4. unscheduled refills, when called in, will be only enough until the next appointment;
5. no use of illegal or street drugs; and
6. random urine drug screens.

When considering issues of drug seeking and compliance, you will discover that you need to ask questions—and sometimes many questions—about the patients' use of their medications when you become suspicious. You will need to become much more comfortable with confrontation in the therapeutic environment.

RESIST EXPANDING BEYOND YOUR AREA OF EXPERTISE

Now that you have the authority to write prescriptions, you may find that you are getting referrals from colleagues who want you to "just write a prescription for my patient." These referrals may come from colleagues you have known for many years. You are going to have to decide how you will handle such requests.

Additionally, requests may come for you to manage or take on new patients who are outside of your established area of expertise. There is temptation to help out in any way that you can. For example, you may have restricted your practice to seeing adults but now you are getting referrals to see children. Perhaps you have not had experience over the past several years with seeing seriously mentally ill patients in your office. Before taking on patients with whom you have had very little experience, you should make every attempt to remain in your area of expertise and try not to become everything for everybody. Keep in mind that adverse events can occur in just about any situation, including those in which you may be trying to help out a friend, family member, colleague, or very good referral source.

SHOULD YOU PRESCRIBE FOR A PATIENT
THAT YOU HAVE NEVER SEEN?

This is a difficult question. It is impossible to design a system in which prescribers do not at times prescribe for patients they have not seen. It will invariably happen that you will want to go out of town for a vacation, conference, or whatever the occasion may be. You will need someone to cover for you while you are away, and you will have to make sure that the person covering for you can indeed handle medications and has the ability to prescribe should the need arise. For example, suppose a patient develops a mild reaction such as itching to a medication you prescribed. It may not be enough simply to tell the patient to discontinue the medication: The patient may need something like diphenhydramine to ease the itch.

Just as you will need someone to cover you, there may be occasions when you will cover for someone else. You may know the person for whom you are covering and feel very comfortable with that colleague. However, if you are part of coverage for a group you may not know some members of the group very well. There may come occasions when you will receive a telephone call from a patient whom you have never met, have never even talked to previously, and for whom you have no medical records available. What do you do?

Here is a little tip that you may find useful. When on call, ask those patients whom you do not know but who are calling for refills to read the information and directions straight from the bottle. That way you can generally find out when the prescription was last filled and whether it is reasonable that the patient would be out of medication at this time. If you are suspicious, ask the patient to read the directions of how to take the medication a second time, this time backwards. If they have the bottle in front of them, it should not be that difficult. If you are still suspicious, you may fill the prescription for a limited number of pills sufficient enough to get the patient until their provider is available again.

So it is probably unrealistic to expect that you will never be called on to prescribe for someone whom you have never met. Be flexible, use common sense, and take care of the patient and yourself.

A FEW FINAL THOUGHTS

After more than 15 years of psychologists prescribing in the U.S. military and almost 5 years of prescribing in Louisiana and New Mexico, psychologists with prescriptive authority continue to prescribe medications safely and effectively. Although opponents of psychologists prescribing (some even within psychology) speculate that psychologists may not be safe prescribers, more than 15 years of evidence—not speculation—indicates otherwise. To date, there have been no complaints filed against medical or prescribing psychologists with regard to prescribing medications.

Having prescriptive authority does indeed open up new avenues to psychologists. Medical and prescribing psychologists have become more of a "one stop shop" for patients, and this has resulted in lower costs to the patient.

They are filling voids in the mental health care system and improving services to those who have found it difficult to access services in the past.

Growing our profession has never been easy or without turmoil. There were those who did not agree with the move from the academic environment to the clinic. There were those who did not approve of psychology providing mental health services after World War II. Dr. George Albee (2000) responded to the training model adopted by clinical psychology by saying, "Psychologists have sold their souls to the devil: the disease model of mental disorders" (p. 248). You can please some of the psychologists some of the time, but you can never please all of the psychologists any of the time. I do believe this change in our profession has been good for psychology, has been good for mental health care, and has been good for the consumers of mental health care.

Is prescriptive authority for you? It may or it may not be. This is a question that each must ask herself or himself. However, it should be a question that you have the choice to ask yourself. We should not deny our colleagues who choose to pursue this line of study the right to do so. In much the same manner as many of our colleagues make choices about pursuing specialty training in neuropsychology, forensics, or rehabilitation psychology, psychopharmacology is a choice that should be available to us. Now it is.

In making your decision, keep in mind that with this added knowledge and skill come added responsibilities. You will have new responsibilities to the patients for whom you prescribe. You will have responsibilities to learn and stay current in an entirely different body of literature. You will be responsible for addressing more after-hour phone calls than perhaps you have in your entire career up to this point. You will be faced with responsibility for patient issues for which you would refer to others in the past. You will have more areas of risk for which you will be liable. Why in the world, then, would you decide to do this?

Out of all the disciplines that now prescribe, psychologists are uniquely positioned to balance humanism with the ability to help resolve, using multiple modalities, some of the misery that can come with the human condition. In sum, training in psychopharmacology is a good thing for all psychologists, whether or not the choice is made to pursue prescriptive authority. This chapter was just a little about the nuts and bolts of prescribing. Just as perhaps our experiences with psychotherapy are not exactly alike, our experiences with prescriptive authority will not be exactly alike either. However, know that medical and prescribing psychologists are making a positive difference in our mental health care system. As the number of psychologists with prescriptive authority grows, so too will the impact on the profession and our patients.

REFERENCES

Albee, G. W. (2000). The Boulder model's fatal flaw. *American Psychologist, 55*, 247–248. doi:10.1037/0003-066X.55.2.247

Ashton, A. K., Jamerson, B. D., Weinstein, W. L., & Wagoner, C. (2005). Antidepressant-related adverse effects impacting treatment compliance: Results of a patient survey. *Current Therapeutic Research, Clinical and Experimental, 66*, 96–106. doi:10.1016/j.curtheres.2005.04.006

Castel, L. D., Williams, K. A., Bosworth, H. B., Eisen, S. V., Hahn, E. A., Irwin, D. E., . . . DeVellis, R. F. (2008). Content validity in the PROMIS social-health domain: A qualitative analysis of focus-group data. *Quality of Life Research, 17*, 737–749. doi:10.1007/s11136-008-9352-3

Cooper, C., Bebbington, P., King, M., Brugha, T., Meltzer, H., Bhugra, D., & Jenkins, R. (2007). Why people do not take their psychotropic drugs as prescribed: Results of the 2000 National Psychiatric Morbidity Survey. *Acta Psychiatrica Scandinavica, 116*, 47–53. doi:10.1111/j.1600-0447.2006.00974.x

Hatfield, D. R., & Ogles, B. M. (2004). The use of outcome measures by psychologists in clinical practice. *Professional Psychology, Research and Practice, 35*, 485–491. doi:10.1037/0735-7028.35.5.485

Munetz, M. R., & Benjamin, S. (1988). How to examine patients using the Abnormal Involuntary Movement Scale. *Hospital & Community Psychiatry, 39*, 1172–1177.

Peck, B. M., Ubel, P. A., Roter, D. L., Goold, S. D., Asch, D. A., Jeffreys, S. A., . . . Tulsk, J. A. (2004). Do unmet expectations for specific tests, referrals, and new medications reduce patients' satisfaction? *Journal of General Internal Medicine, 19*, 1080–1087. doi:10.1111/j.1525-1497.2004.30436.x

5

ETHICAL CONSIDERATIONS IN PHARMACOTHERAPY FOR PSYCHOLOGISTS

ROBERT E. McGRATH AND BETH N. ROM-RYMER

What are the psychologist's professional responsibilities to the patient who is taking psychotropic medications? To what extent do the responsibilities differ if the psychologist is a prescriber versus a provider of psychotherapy? Are those responsibilities consistent with traditional standards of professional practice that have evolved to govern the activities of psychologists as psychotherapists and consultants, or are there unique responsibilities related to pharmacotherapy? These questions become more important as the number of patients who receive medication and psychologists' involvement in pharmacotherapy increase.

In this chapter, we first discuss the three levels of pharmacotherapy involvement that psychologists can attain. Next, we describe the evolution of psychology practice guidelines that deal with ethics in pharmacotherapy. Finally, we discuss some ethical issues specific to the psychologist involved in pharmacotherapy.

THREE LEVELS OF INVOLVEMENT IN PHARMACOTHERAPY

As background to answering critical ethical questions such as those posed in the first paragraph of this chapter, it is important to describe the various roles that psychologists may play in the treatment of an individual who is taking psychotropic medications. The triadic model of training in pharmacotherapy first suggested by Smyer et al. (1993), and described in Chapter 2 of this volume, can be generalized to provide a framework for a psychologist's level of involvement in pharmacotherapy. Specifically, the level of a psychologist's involvement in the pharmacotherapy of their patients can be conceptualized as a dimension on which three stop points can be easily identified. At one end of the spectrum are psychologists who prescribe. It is the quest for prescriptive authority that has raised consciousness about psychologists' involvement in pharmacotherapy, and it has been estimated that more than 1,500 psychologists have completed the didactic portion of Level 3 training (Ax, Fagan, & Resnick, 2009), but only about 100 psychologists are currently prescribing in the agencies and states where it is permitted. Many more psychologists are already operating at lower levels of involvement in pharmacotherapy. A lower level of involvement, consistent with Level 2 training, occurs when the psychologist plays a role in medication decision making whereas another individual, usually a member of another profession with prescriptive authority, maintains legal responsibility for the final choice. VandenBos and Williams (2000) found that 7% of psychologists who responded to their survey reported they were involved in medication decision making for half or more of their patients. American Psychological Association (APA) policy has considered such collaboration within the scope of psychological practice since 1981 (APA Board of Professional Affairs, 1981), and the best accounting suggests that to date 17 state licensing boards have formally recognized psychologists' authority to participate in some way in the medication decision-making process (http://www.division55.org/wiki/index.php?title=Medication_Consultation_Opinions), offering an additional level of legal protection for psychologists collaborating in those jurisdictions.

Finally, Level 1 training (basic familiarity) is consistent with the recognition that pharmacotherapy is a given in clinical practice. For example, VandenBos and Williams (2000) found that 95% of psychologists reported they work in settings where medications are "routinely" used, and on average 43% of patients being seen by psychologists were receiving medications. With such widespread use, it is not surprising that psychologists regularly discuss issues surrounding pharmacotherapy with patients and their physicians. However, in most cases this interaction involves providing information and supportive services rather than active involvement in the decision-making process.

EVOLUTION OF PRACTICE GUIDELINES

The question of whether traditional standards of practice in psychology are sufficient to our increasing involvement in pharmacotherapy was first broached by Buelow and Chafetz (1996). They concluded that additional ethical standards specific to prescribing were appropriate, though the range of topics covered in their discussion was fairly narrow and somewhat generic:

- Psychologists should only prescribe after an appropriate psychological assessment. They believed this standard should be considered inviolate even in emergency situations.
- Treatment should always be based on informed consent.
- Prescribing psychologists should choose the best course of treatment, including consideration of the cost–benefit ratio for each treatment, but they should prefer psychosocial over biological interventions.
- Psychologists should avoid polypharmacy and strive to develop the simplest drug treatment regimen possible.
- Prescribing psychologists should exercise special care when treating the medically ill.
- Prescribing psychologists should be sensitive to the potential for adverse events.

The next detailed analysis of changes in practice standards was generated by McGrath et al. (2004). Like Buelow and Chafetz (1996), McGrath et al. focused on a more specific set of issues, including the following:

- ensuring that prescribers maintain their professional identity as psychologists (McGrath et al. concluded that the postdoctoral requirement for advanced training in psychopharmacology was essential to achieving this goal; for a different perspective, see Ax et al., 2009);
- development of a psychological model of prescribing;
- legal issues for psychologists involved in pharmacotherapy in jurisdictions without prescriptive authority;
- minimizing the use of brief office visits in prescriptive practice;
- consideration of psychosocial alternatives in prescriptive practice;
- interactions with the pharmaceutical industry;
- interactions with other professionals and facility staff; and
- continuing education requirements.

The next important step in describing optimal practice in pharmacotherapy began with a discussion in 2004 within the leadership of APA Division 55 (American Society for the Advancement of Pharmacotherapy) about the need for more formal guidelines concerning the implications of increasing involvement in pharmacotherapy for professional practice. Several factors spurred this discussion. Psychologists had begun prescribing in larger numbers, and the use of psychotropic medications was continuing to grow. The length of psychiatric visits was continuing to decline (Olfson, Marcus, & Pincus, 1999), and concerns were expressed about psychologists moving down the same path (e.g., McGrath, 2004). One factor in particular that was rapidly evolving was public and professional concern about the role the pharmaceutical industry plays in prescribing practices. There was an interest in reinforcing Smyer et al.'s (1993) conclusions about the importance of continuing education regardless of level of involvement in pharmacotherapy. Finally, a formal discussion of optimal practice in pharmacotherapy was considered valuable as a demonstration that psychologists took the gravity of prescribing very seriously.

In response to these discussions, Beth Rom-Rymer, who served as the president of the division at the time, appointed a task force to look into the question of ethical standards in pharmacotherapy. Members of the task force included the first author of this chapter as chair, prescribing psychologists, representatives of training programs, and a liaison from Division 18 (Psychologists in Public Service) of the APA. One of the first conclusions was that the development of distinct ethical standards was probably premature given the early state of prescriptive authority in psychology, especially because ethical standards are legally binding for licensed psychologists through their incorporation into licensing laws and regulations.

A second option would have involved an essay on the implications of the existing ethical standards for pharmacotherapy. This was the course adopted by the American Psychiatric Association (2009), which publishes an annotated version of the *Principles of Medical Ethics* specifically focusing on ethical standards for psychiatrists. Instead, the task force chose a path more common in professional psychology, which involves the drafting of what are known as practice guidelines.

In APA parlance, practice guidelines are distinct from treatment guidelines and ethical standards. Treatment guidelines provide recommendations for clinical interventions that are usually specific to a certain disorder, method of treatment, or both (APA, 2002a); treatment guidelines may be developed for cognitive-behavioral treatment or for the treatment of depression, for example. Practice guidelines and ethical standards differ from treatment guidelines in that they have to do with general professional conduct in a particular domain of psychological practice.

Practice guidelines differ from ethical standards in that the latter are mandatory and may be accompanied by an enforcement mechanism. Practice guidelines are aspirational in intent, intended to facilitate the continued systematic development of the profession and to help encourage a high level of professional practice by psychologists. They are not intended to be mandatory or exhaustive and may not be applicable to every professional or in every clinical situation.

Once the format of the product was determined, the task force went to work developing specific guidelines. These went through numerous rounds of review and revision, and as of August 2009 were accepted by the APA Council of Representatives as official policy of the association. The current version of the document (APA Council of Representatives, 2009), titled *Guidelines Regarding Psychologists' Involvement in Pharmacological Issues*, represents the most detailed consideration of the implications of pharmacotherapy for psychological practice completed to date. It consists of 17 guidelines of varying relevance to the three levels of involvement in pharmacotherapy. The guidelines and the levels of involvement to which each applies may be found in Table 5.1.

Several general points can be made about the guidelines. First, the articulation between guideline and professional activities is an important one. Some principles are applicable regardless of the psychologist's level of involvement in the process of pharmacotherapy, though the implications of the principle vary across contexts. Other principles are specifically relevant to the prescribing psychologist, or to psychologists involved in the decision-making process. Second, the guidelines were worded in a manner to reinforce their aspirational intent. A good deal of effort was required to rid the principles of any implication of mandated action. This goal seems to have been met when one reader noted that the guidelines had the phrasing of educational rather than legal principles. Third, the guidelines are divided into general principles that should be considered in any situation involving pharmacotherapy; and principles specifically relevant to education, assessment, intervention and consultation, and professional relationships.

Though the guidelines do not represent distinct standards and are intended to spell out some of the implications of the APA Ethics Code (APA, 2002b; http://www.apa.org/ethics/code/code.pdf) psychologists' involvement in pharmacotherapy, there are a number of issues addressed that are distinctly relevant to the setting in which patients are receiving medications. The rest of this chapter focuses on several issues that are uniquely relevant in the context of pharmacotherapy, or for which psychologists' traditional practices merit modification in this context.

ISSUE 1: WHAT SHOULD PSYCHOLOGISTS KNOW ABOUT MEDICATIONS?

For the prescribing psychologist, state law or regulation usually defines a legal minimum, though a prescriber might believe education in excess of the legally mandated minimum is appropriate. For all other psychologists, the

TABLE 5.1
List of Guidelines

Guideline	Relevant activities		
	Prescribing	Collaborating	Providing information
General			
1. Psychologists are encouraged to consider objectively the scope of their competence in pharmacotherapy and to seek consultation as appropriate before offering recommendations about psychotropic medications.	X	X	X
2. Psychologists are urged to evaluate their own feelings and attitudes about the role of medication in the treatment of psychological disorders, as these feelings and attitudes can potentially affect communications with patients.	X	X	X
3. Psychologists involved in prescribing or collaborating are sensitive to the developmental, age and aging, educational, sex and gender, language, health status, and cultural–ethnicity factors that can moderate the interpersonal and biological aspects of pharmacotherapy relevant to the populations they serve.	X	X	
Education			
4. Psychologists are urged to identify a level of knowledge concerning pharmacotherapy for the treatment of psychological disorders that is appropriate to the populations they serve and the type of practice they wish to establish, and to engage in educational experiences as appropriate to achieve and maintain that level of knowledge.	X	X	X
5. Psychologists strive to be sensitive to the potential for adverse effects associated with the psychotropic medications used by their patients.	X	X	X
6. Psychologists involved in prescribing or collaborating are encouraged to familiarize themselves with the technological resources that can enhance decision making during the course of treatment.	X	X	

TABLE 5.1
List of Guidelines   *(Continued)*

Guideline	Relevant activities		
	Prescribing	Collaborating	Providing information
Assessment			
7. Psychologists with prescriptive authority strive to familiarize themselves with key procedures for monitoring the physical and psychological sequelae of the medications used to treat psychological disorders, including laboratory examinations and overt signs of adverse or unintended effects.	X		
8. Psychologists with prescriptive authority regularly strive to monitor the physiological status of the patients they treat with medication, particularly when there is a physical condition that might complicate the response to psychotropic medication or predispose a patient to experience an adverse reaction.	X		
9. Psychologists are encouraged to explore issues surrounding patient adherence and feelings about medication.	X	X	X
Intervention and consultation			
10. Psychologists are urged to develop a relationship that will allow the populations they serve to feel comfortable exploring issues surrounding medication use.	X	X	X
11. To the extent deemed appropriate, psychologists involved in prescribing or collaboration adopt a biopsychosocial approach to case formulation that considers both psychosocial and biological factors.	X	X	
12. The psychologist with prescriptive authority is encouraged to use an expanded informed consent process to incorporate additional issues specific to prescribing.	X		
13. When making decisions about the use of psychological treatments, pharmacotherapy, or their combination, the psychologist with prescriptive authority considers the best interests of the patient, current research, and when appropriate, the needs of the community.	X		

(continues)

TABLE 5.1
List of Guidelines *(Continued)*

	Relevant activities		
Guideline	Prescribing	Collaborating	Providing information
14. Psychologists involved in prescribing or collaborating strive to be sensitive to the subtle influences of effective marketing on professional behavior and the potential for bias in information in their clinical decisions about the use of medications.	X	X	
15. Psychologists with prescriptive authority are encouraged to use interactions with the patient surrounding the act of prescribing to learn more about the patient's characteristic patterns of interpersonal behavior.	X		
Relationships			
16. Psychologists with prescriptive authority are sensitive to maintaining appropriate relationships with other providers of psychological services.	X		
17. Psychologists are urged to maintain appropriate relationships with providers of biological interventions.	X	X	X

Note. From *Guidelines regarding psychologists' involvement in pharmacological issues* (pp. 51–52), by the American Psychological Association Division 55 Task Force on Practice Guidelines, 2009, Washington, DC: Author. Copyright 2009 by the American Psychological Association.

level of ongoing training appropriate in pharmacotherapy remains at the psychologist's discretion. Guideline 4 calls for psychologists to consider what level of education about pharmacotherapy would be appropriate for the populations they serve and the nature of their practice. To our knowledge, this is the first practice document accepted by the association that has explicitly encouraged all practicing psychologists to consider this question.[1] It suggests that psychologists should consider whether it is in their patients' best interests for them to become more active as advocates for optimal care, even though other professionals are ultimately responsible for decisions.

[1] Smyer et al. (1993), who were focused primarily on training, recommended continuing education for all psychologists in pharmacotherapy, a recommendation that led to adoption of a regulation in the state of Georgia for all licensed psychologists to complete 3 hours of continuing education in psychopharmacology every 2 years. However, that recommendation was never incorporated into any documents that focused on guidelines for practice.

Factors that may play a role in these considerations include the following:

- *The proportion of patients who are taking psychotropic medications.* Many psychologists work in settings where most if not all patients receive medications. Additional training in medication management can be particularly cost-effective in settings that cater to members of a population where a certain class of medications (e.g., opiates in a pain management clinic) is commonly prescribed.
- *The severity of side effects associated with those medications.* The psychologist often has more contact with the patient than any other provider. This means the psychologist can serve a central role in the monitoring of life-threatening adverse events, but only if the psychologist is sensitized to the markers for those events.
- *The age and medical complexity of those patients who are taking medications.* These factors contribute to the risks associated with the use of psychotropic medications. Psychologists who work in settings that specialize in the treatment of the very young, the older population, or individuals with medical complications can play a particularly important role in ensuring patient safety.
- *The effectiveness with which patients advocate for themselves.* This can be moderated by various factors, including cultural differences in dealing with the doctor–patient relationship (Rey, 2006), understanding of health and health services ("health literacy"; U.S. Department of Health and Human Services, 2000), and various other factors.
- *Their perception of the quality of pharmacological care provided to patients in the settings where they serve.* Most prescriptions for psychotropic medications are not written by psychiatric specialists (Pincus et al., 1998). Even when psychiatric care is available, the brevity of psychiatric appointments (Olfson et al., 1999) can undermine optimal care for patients with more complex circumstances. The psychologist can help compensate for the shortage in access to specialized psychiatric care even in the absence of prescriptive authority.

Guideline 4 also raises questions about the extent to which patients would benefit from additional training for psychologists in clinical medicine, particularly the recognition of pseudopsychiatric conditions because of illness or medication such as pediatric autoimmune neuropsychiatric disorders associated with streptococcal infections (PANDAS), hyper- and hypothyroidism, and steroid-induced psychosis. Given the multiple variables relevant to deciding whether and to what extent additional training in psychopharmacology would enhance patient care, no single standard can be offered for the amount and type of such training that would be appropriate or even whether additional training in psychopharmacology is called for. The guideline simply encourages psychologists to consider the question. (For further discussion of this topic, see Barnett & Neel, 2000.)

ISSUE 2: WHAT IS THE PSYCHOLOGICAL MODEL OF PRESCRIBING?

Several of the guidelines have implications for the emergence of a uniquely psychological model of prescribing. Most directly relevant is Guideline 11, which calls for a biopsychosocial approach to prescribing or collaboration. This term has been widely adopted among the health care professions, so it is important to consider whether psychologists will mean something different when they use this term in the context of pharmacotherapy. The commentary that accompanies the guideline suggests psychologists can and should strive for a unique understanding of the integrationist model of patient care, an understanding that is nicely captured in the concept of a "psychobiosocial" model as described by LeVine and Foster (see Chapter 6, this volume).

Although many disciplines espouse a biopsychosocial model, the term is often used to refer to a treatment approach where psychosocial approaches are adjunctive to the biological treatment and may even be used only to enhance cooperation with the biological treatment. For the psychologist, the model instead calls for consideration of cultural, biological, educational, psychological, and social factors in every step of the treatment. Furthermore, because psychosocial interventions are associated with fewer side effects, there should be a bias in favor of the former treatments, particularly in those circumstances where research is finding advantages to the use of psychosocial (e.g., Antonuccio, Danton, DeNelsky, Greenberg, & Gordon, 1999; Bartels et al., 2002; Brown et al, 2008; Casacalenda, Perry, & Looper, 2002; Fabiano et al., 2007) or combined treatment (Pediatric OCD Treatment Team, 2004; The Treatment of Adolescent Depression Study Team, 2004; Walkup et al., 2008) over biological interventions alone.

This guideline is also intended to combat pressures to reduce the quality of treatment that are often associated with an exclusive focus on pharmacotherapy as the treatment of choice. The prescribing psychologist who works from a true biopsychosocial model is going to use brief medication visits with discretion, even when the patient is referred specifically for medication consultation by another mental health provider. As Ally pointed out (see Chapter 4, this volume), psychologists will find themselves prescribing in situations in which they have no history with the patient, and perhaps they are required to act quickly to deal with an emergency situation. Even then, psychologists are expected to operate as psychologists first and prescribers second, considering the patient in a broader context than immediate relief. Guideline 15 notes that in circumstances where treatment begins with a primarily biological intervention, the patient's style of response to that intervention can provide an important avenue into the exploration of more psychosocial issues.

Guideline 12 is also related to this broader understanding of the practice of pharmacotherapy. The parameters of informed consent expand substantially when both biological and psychosocial interventions are under consideration. The guideline is accompanied by a checklist of 16 issues that may be important in this context. Examples include providing information about the agent recommended and the rationale for its choice, describing both the potential benefits and risks of the protocol and how to control for the latter, estimating the duration and cost of treatment and the time to therapeutic effect, reviewing the risks associated with sudden discontinuation of the medication, discussing assessment procedures associated with the intervention, and providing patient education in a format understandable by the patient. The goal is to help the patient develop a sense as a collaborator in the treatment decision-making process rather than the simple recipient of the prescriber's decisions. All of this must be accomplished with an understanding of the patient's personal and culture-based beliefs about the doctor–patient relationship and the use of medications, as well as their capacity to participate in the process.

ISSUE 3: HOW SHALL WE DEAL WITH PHARMACEUTICAL MARKETING?

The guidelines provide a detailed description of the various ways the pharmaceutical industry attempts to influence medication decision making, with particular emphasis on the role of the pharmaceutical industry in the control of information about the efficacy and safety of medications (see also Chapter 7, this volume).[2]

Perhaps the most extensively discussed subtle influence on medication decision making has been gift giving. It has been suggested that gifts contribute to overvaluation of the medication through the creation of cognitive

---

[2]It should be noted that most of the research described in this section has been conducted with family physicians or other generalists. The extent to which the influences described apply to specialty practitioners such as psychiatrists and prescribing psychologists is largely unknown and represents an important external validity issue.

dissonance (e.g., Chimonas, Brennan, & Rothman, 2007). As a result, both health care organizations and pharmaceutical companies have placed restrictions on the value of gifts in recent years, yet the rising use of medications has continued unabated. This pattern suggests that the importance of gift giving as an influence on decision making may well have been overestimated, and the more important factors are more subtle. Drug representatives try to establish a personal relationship with the prescriber, and such a relationship is probably more likely to create a motivation to think well of the representative's product line than anything as blatant as a gift. I (Rom-Rymer) personally witnessed another example of these subtle influences when a colleague of mine, a family physician, was hired by a drug company to "educate" other physicians about a certain medication over dinner. My colleague was pleased with the restrictions built into the event that seemed intended to minimize its influence on the recipients of the talk, including the absence of drug representatives and limited mention of the sponsor. When I pointed out that the evening might also have been intended to convince him of the efficacy of the medication, he gave up lecturing for the drug company.

The commentary that accompanies the guideline describes several of these subtle influences. One was labeled the *principle of least effort* by Haug (1997), the tendency for physicians to balance time demands and the need for information by relying on easily available sources of information, even if they know the source is of low quality, over more authoritative but less easily accessible sources of information. A good recent example of this principle in action that has actually been to the detriment of the pharmaceutical industry has to do with the black box warning on suicidal ideation associated with use of antidepressants in children and adolescents. A recent survey (Cordero, Rudd, Bryan, & Corso, 2008) found that over 90% of primary care physicians who responded believe the black box warning referred to an increased risk of death by suicide. The finding suggests that most physicians have never read the black box warning but are instead relying on the popular press or other sources even though the actual warning is readily available to them. To the extent that the pharmaceutical industry is able to influence popular sources of information, the industry is able to influence what physicians believe about medications, at least in the population of primary care providers that prescribe the vast majority of psychotropic medications.

We continue to learn about the various methods that can be used to influence physicians' prescribing practices (for a summary, see Fugh-Berman & Ahari, 2007). Ultimately, the importance of these factors may pale in comparison to the pharmaceutical industry's control over what information is published (see Chapter 7, this volume), but they can contribute to prescribers coming to believe a medication is more effective than it actually is. In this way, medication decision making can be subtly influenced without the prescriber experiencing a sense of being manipulated. It is hoped that psychologists' sensitivity to issues of cognitive error and personal influence will help them to avoid the practices that have tarnished the reputation of medicine and the pharmaceutical industry.

ISSUE 4: HOW WILL PROFESSIONAL RELATIONSHIPS CHANGE?

Prescribing, and even active collaboration, creates the potential for a dramatic shift in psychologists' role within the health care system. As the doctoral-level profession with the most extensive training in how to talk with patients about even uncomfortable topics, enhanced training in both the biological and psychosocial interventions, and our comfort dealing with both emotional disorders and the behavioral aspects of medical treatment, psychologists have tremendous potential as contributors to the system. In fact, psychologists who remain true to their roots can fill an essential niche in the health care system, by becoming advocates of integrated care and the patient's primary advisor. This exciting new possibility, as the professional best positioned to serve as the treatment coordinator for individuals with emotional, behavioral, or both issues associated with their medical treatment, merits serious consideration as important to improving both the status of psychology and the quality of health care services.

It will be important for psychologists to consider seriously the changes prescriptive authority will bring to their professional relationships. Increasingly, psychologists will serve as consultants to other health care professionals and even to other mental health providers. As outlined in Guidelines 16 and 17, psychologists must be ready for these changing roles and accept the new possibilities but also the new risks attendant with those changes.

CONCLUSION

The guidelines represent the most detailed discussion of the implications of pharmacotherapy for psychological practice to date, but they represent only a starting point. As psychologists continue to increase their involvement in pharmacotherapy through prescriptive authority, and ultimately through a larger presence in primary care settings, psychologists will continue to struggle to define mandatory and optimal practices in those settings. Our involvement in prescribing and our increasing involvement in pharmacotherapy, in general, creates an opportunity to improve the quality of pharmacological care for individuals with psychological disorders. We must take advantage of that opportunity for the good of the individuals that we serve.

REFERENCES

American Psychiatric Association. (2009). *The principles of medical ethics with annotations especially applicable to psychiatry* (2009 ed.). Arlington, VA: Author.

American Psychological Association. (2002a). Criteria for practice guideline development and evaluation. *American Psychologist, 57,* 1048–1051. doi:10.1037/0003-066X.57.12.1048

American Psychological Association. (2002b). Ethical principles of psychologists and code of conduct. *American Psychologist, 57,* 1060–1073.

American Psychological Association Board of Professional Affairs. (1981). *Task force report: Psychologists' use of physical interventions.* Washington, DC: American Psychological Association.

American Psychological Association Council of Representatives. (2009). *Guidelines regarding psychologists' involvement in pharmacological issues.* Washington, DC: Author.

Antonuccio, D. O., Danton, W. G., DeNelsky, G. Y., Greenberg, R. P., & Gordon, J. S. (1999). Raising questions about antidepressants. *Psychotherapy and Psychosomatics, 68,* 3–14. doi:10.1159/000012304

Ax, R. K., Fagan, T. J., & Resnick, R. J. (2009). Predoctoral prescriptive authority training: The rationale and a combined model. *Psychological Services, 6,* 85–95. doi:10.1037/a0013824

Barnett, J. E., & Neel, M. L. (2000). Must all psychologists study psychopharmacology? *Professional Psychology, Research and Practice, 31,* 619–627. doi:10.1037/0735-7028.31.6.619

Bartels, S. J., Dums, A. R., Oxman, T. E., Schneider, L. S., Arean, P. A., Alexopoulos, G. S., & Jeste, D. V. (2002). Evidence-based practices in geriatric mental health care. *Psychiatric Services (Washington, DC), 53,* 1419–1431. doi:10.1176/appi.ps.53.11.1419

Brown, R. T., Antonuccio, D. O., DuPaul, G. J., Fristad, M. E., King, C. E., Leslie, L. K., . . . Vitiello, B. (2008). *Childhood mental health disorders: Evidence base and contextual factors for psychosocial, psychopharmacological, and combined interventions.* Washington, DC: American Psychological Association. doi:10.1037/11638-000

Buelow, G. D., & Chafetz, M. D. (1996). Proposed ethical practice guidelines for clinical pharmacopsychology: Sharpening a new focus in psychology. *Professional Psychology, Research and Practice, 27,* 53–58. doi:10.1037/0735-7028.27.1.53

Casacalenda, N., Perry, J. C., & Looper, K. (2002). Remission in major depressive disorder: A comparison of pharmacotherapy, psychotherapy, and control conditions. *The American Journal of Psychiatry, 159,* 1354–1360. doi:10.1176/appi.ajp.159.8.1354

Chimonas, S., Brennan, T. A., & Rothman, D. J. (2007). Physicians and drug representatives: Exploring the dynamics of the relationship. *Journal of General Internal Medicine, 22,* 184–190. doi:10.1007/s11606-006-0041-z

Cordero, L., Rudd, M. D., Bryan, C. J., & Corso, K. A. (2008). Accuracy of primary care medical providers' understanding of the FDA black box warning label for antidepressants. *Primary Care & Community Psychiatry, 13,* 109–114.

Fabiano, G. A., Pelham, W. E., Jr., Gnagy, E. M., Burrows-MacLean, L., Coles, E. K., Chacko, A., . . . Robb, J. A. (2007). The single and combined effects of multiple intensities of behavior modification and methylphenidate for children with attention deficit hyperactivity disorder in a classroom setting. *School Psychology Review, 36,* 195–216.

Fugh-Berman, A., & Ahari, S. (2007). Following the script: How drug reps make friends and influence doctors. *PLoS Medicine, 4,* 621–625. doi:10.1371/journal. pmed.0040150

Haug, J. D. (1997). Physicians' preferences for information sources: A meta-analytic study. *Bulletin of the Medical Library Association, 85,* 223–232.

McGrath, R. E. (2004). Saving our psychosocial souls. *American Psychologist, 59,* 644–645. doi:10.1037/0003-066X.59.7.644

McGrath, R. E., Wiggins, J. G., Sammons, M. T., Levant, R. F., Brown, A., & Stock, W. (2004). Professional issues in pharmacotherapy for psychologists. *Professional Psychology: Research and Practice, 35,* 158–163. doi:10.1037/0735-7028.35.2.158

Olfson, M., Marcus, S. C., & Pincus, H. A. (1999). Trends in office-based psychiatric practice. *The American Journal of Psychiatry, 156,* 451–457.

Pediatric OCD Treatment Team. (2004). Cognitive-behavior therapy, sertraline, and their combination for children and adolescents with obsessive-compulsive disorder: The pediatric OCD treatment study (POTS) randomized controlled trial. *JAMA, 292,* 1969–1976. doi:10.1001/jama.292.16.1969

Pincus, H. A., Tanielian, T. L., Marcus, S. C., Olfson, M., Zarin, D. A., Thompson, J., & Zito, J. M. (1998). Prescribing trends in psychotropic medications: Primary care, psychiatry, and other medical specialties. *JAMA, 279,* 526–531. doi:10.1001/jama.279.7.526

Rey, J. A. (2006). Interface of multiculturalism in psychopharmacology. *Journal of Pharmacy Practice, 19,* 379–385. doi:10.1177/0897190007300734

Smyer, M. A., Balster, R. L., Egli, D., Johnson, D. L., Kilbey, M. M., Leith, N. J., & Puente, A. E. (1993). Summary of the report of the ad hoc task force on psychopharmacology of the American Psychological Association. *Professional Psychology, Research and Practice, 24,* 394–403. doi:10.1037/0735-7028.24.4.394

The Treatment of Adolescent Depression Study Team. (2004). Fluoxetine, cognitive-behavioral therapy, and their combination for adolescents with depression: Treatment for Adolescents with Depression Study (TADS) randomized controlled trial. *JAMA, 292,* 807–820. doi:10.1001/jama.292.7.807

U.S. Department of Health and Human Services. (2000). *Healthy People 2010: Understanding and improving health* (2nd ed.). Washington, DC: U.S. Government Printing Office.

VandenBos, G. R., & Williams, S. (2000). Is psychologists' involvement in the prescribing of psychotropic medication really a new activity? *Professional Psychology, Research and Practice, 31*, 615–618. doi:10.1037/0735-7028.31.6.615

Walkup, J. T., Albano, A. M., Piacentini, J., Birmaher, B., Compton, S. N., Sherrill, J. T., . . . Kendall, P. C. (2008). Cognitive behavioral therapy, sertraline, or a combination in childhood anxiety. *The New England Journal of Medicine, 359*, Article 10.1056/NEJMoa0804633.

6

INTEGRATION OF PSYCHOTHERAPY AND PHARMACOTHERAPY BY PRESCRIBING–MEDICAL PSYCHOLOGISTS: A PSYCHOBIOSOCIAL MODEL OF CARE

ELAINE S. LEVINE AND ELAINE ORABONA FOSTER

The emergence in the 1980s of new psychotropics with a relatively safer side-effect profile led many practitioners and consumers to conclude that the preferred method of treatment for mental disorders was psychotropically based. Subsequent to this enhanced belief in medical management of mental disorders, case studies began to emerge in the clinical literature that led to disparate conclusions about the relative effectiveness of psychotherapy, psychotropics, and combined treatment. Fortunately, within the last 15 years, empirical studies and meta-analyses have emerged that are clarifying this issue.

An often quoted survey conducted by Consumer Reports in 1994 concluded that people who received psychotherapy were generally pleased with the experience, and their satisfaction was unrelated to the type of treatment or the addition of medication (Hollon, 1995). Outcome studies regarding children, adolescents, and adults are now available. Walkup et al. (2008) reported that cognitive behavioral therapy (CBT) or sertraline reduced the severity of anxiety in children with anxiety disorders, and a combination of the two interventions led to superior results. The 3-year follow-up of a multimodal treatment study of children with attention-deficit/hyperactivity disorder (ADHD) indicated an early advantage to a medication and long-term benefits for psychotherapy in the amelioration of psychological and psychosocial symptoms associated with the disorder (Jensen et al., 2007). In adolescent depression research, the well-designed Treatment for Adolescents with Depression Study reported that, at 36 weeks, similar remission rates were achieved for the fluoxetine (55%), CBT (64%), and combined treatment (60%) groups. It is important to note that those with combined treatment remitted earlier (Kennard et al., 2009). Hollon et al. (2005) conducted an extensive review of the literature from 1980 to 2004 to compare the relative efficacy of medications and psychotherapy alone and in combination in the treatment of depression among the adult and geriatric populations. Hollon et al. concluded that medication typically led to rapid and robust effects and prevented symptom return so long as continued. Interpersonal psychotherapy and CBT were equally as effective in acute phases as medication. It is important to note that the gains of CBT appeared more likely to endure following termination. Other studies that used specific outcome measures have demonstrated that combination therapy can decrease relapse rates (Hogarty, 1993); improve medication adherence (Goodwin & Jamison, 2007); reduce readmission rates (Perlick, Rosenheck, Clarkin, Sirey, & Raue, 1999); increase motivation and psychological mindedness (de Jonghe, Kool, van Aalst, Dekker, & Peen, 2001); and reduce dropout rate compared with psychotherapy alone (Pampallona, Bollini, & Tibaldi, 2004). Despite recent research that demonstrated the efficacy of combined treatments, Olfson and Marcus's (2009) review of the Medical Expenditures Panel Surveys of 1966 and of 2005 revealed that antidepressant medications are the most commonly prescribed class of medications in the United States, and individuals treated with antidepressants were more likely to also receive treatment with antipsychotics and less likely to undergo psychotherapy. Low rates of any treatment among racial or ethnic minorities have persisted.

The impetus for psychologists to prescribe has been propelled by a recognition of the critical need to increase access to care and the potential benefits of an integrative, pharmacotherapy approach. Therefore, it is incumbent on psychologists to develop a systematic approach to that integration. The strategic integration of psychotherapy and pharmacotherapy by prescribing–medical psychologists is an evolutionary approach to addressing the critical and increasing mental health needs of U.S. citizens. Combined psychotherapy and pharmacotherapy approaches integrate etiological analysis and treatment strategies based on biological, psychological, and sociological factors often encapsulated in the term *biopsychosocial model of care* (Engel, 1977). It is argued in this chapter that, because of their psychological training, prescribing–medical psychologists can apply the analysis of biological, social, and psychological etiologies and treatment strategies from a somewhat unique framework we call the "psychobiosocial model of care." In the psychobiosocial model posited herein, the therapist–patient relationship and the patient's phenomenological view of psychotherapy and medication management are central. Patient-specific resiliency and vulnerability factors are analyzed within each sphere of functioning. By assessing resilience and vulnerability within all dimensions of functioning, the psychobiosocial model places patient's perceptions, personal values, and needs as the basis for deciding all forms of biological, psychological, and social interventions.

We, both of us being prescribing–medical psychologists, have analyzed our own practices in an effort to elucidate the core elements in which the practice of psychotherapy and pharmacotherapy are combined by those whose core training is as psychologists. The common elements emerging from our approaches were combined in an effort to construct and propose a unique, psychologically based model built on psychologists' unique training. If successful, this model should lead to treatment that can be replicated thereby serving as a framework for evidence-based research. Ideally, a refined model for prescribing–medical psychologists will help foster the evolution of quality, accessible, and integrated mental health care.

COMPONENTS OF A PSYCHOBIOSOCIAL MODEL OF CARE

The psychobiosocial model presented here is based on three major tenets. The first tenet is that psychologists, by virtue of their unique training, offer a specialized skill set for addressing mental health concerns. In their initial training, psychologists are well studied in aspects of behavioral change as well as the biological sciences. Education and training for prescriptive authority adds an additional skill set to an existing diagnostic and treatment armamentarium. Because these skills are taught through specialized programs for psychologists, who have already been trained in human development and the behavioral and cognitive components of psychopathology, they can practice differently, integrating the medication into the therapy process and using medications only when psychotherapy alone is not sufficient to improve functioning.

The second tenet is a result of psychologists' specialized training. Because psychologists are skilled in a broad range of therapeutic intervention techniques, they can help the patient choose the least invasive treatment while focusing on an empirically supported approach as a first-line intervention. When empirical research indicates that psychotropic intervention is efficacious, psychologists recommend this additional treatment to the psychotherapeutic regimen with extensive informed consent, including standard education on indications, risks, benefits, average time-to-therapeutic effect, alternatives, and side-effect profiles of each treatment. The information provided is tailored to the patient, particularly information addressing side effects that are relevant to the patient's concerns, such as weight loss or gain, sleep difficulties, or triglyceride levels. The premise is that the psychologist acts as a consultant to the patient who, with occasional exception (e.g., when frankly psychotic or demented), is considered capable of making an informed decision and who is expected to remain an active problem solver throughout the treatment partnership.

The third tenet has many ramifications. It is postulated that a critical component of the psychologist's psychobiosocial model of care is the integration of the meaning, impact, and usefulness of continued psychotropic medication across the various phases of the therapy process. Although these phases are given different labels across psychotherapeutic models, they will be referred to here as *diagnosis, relationship building, active working, generalization*, and *termination*. We propose that the phases evolve in a hierarchical fashion across the therapeutic process. For example, the diagnostic and relationship phases emerge first but continue to evolve over time. The active-working phase, in which the psychologist and patient embark on systematic interventions to increase resilience by improving adaptability, acquiring new skills, and enhancing physical, psychological, and social functioning, all are shaped by the diagnosis and relationship. Generalization occurs when new cognitions, learning, and behaviors are transferred to new situations as well as to the patient's everyday life. Once enacted, the diagnostic, relationship-building, active-working, and generalization phases continue in a synergistic fashion. The termination phase occurs last, as it involves strategies for ending the psychotherapy, pharmacotherapy, or both, or strategies for long-term maintenance. However, even when termination issues are the focus, diagnosis and relationship building continues, and there may be a return to some active working and generalization to fully prepare the patient for completion or maintenance of treatment. These phases and their relationships with each other are outlined in Figure 6.1.

The following section explicates the means by which psychotherapy and psychopharmacology are integrated in each phase. Patient-specific resiliency and vulnerability are a part of the analysis at each phase. For instance, a specific patient may suffer from a genetic vulnerability, such as a family history of hypertension; however, biological resiliency may be augmented by restricting salt, exercising, and maintaining an ideal body weight. Similarly, a patient's health may be vulnerable to social factors, such as overcrowding or a lack of informal support systems, and resilience may be enhanced by participation in community-based faith groups, volunteer opportunities, or relocation.

The precepts of the model are explicated so they can be used systematically by the prescribing–medical psychologists and, to some degree, by psychologists trained in psychopharmacology without prescriptive authority who nevertheless consult with their patients about medication. The applicability and goodness of fit of the model are then explored by applying the precepts to several current issues in psychopharmacology.

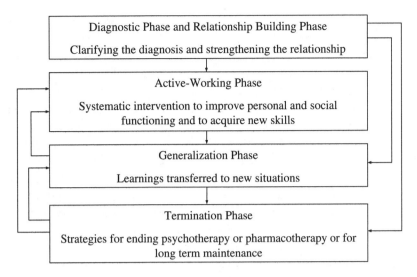

Figure 6.1. Outline of the phases of therapy.

Diagnosis Phase

In the psychobiosocial model, a dynamic orientation toward diagnosis begins concomitant with the establishment of the therapeutic relationship and continues throughout the therapy process. Core elements of effective diagnoses in the psychobiosocial model are outlined in Exhibit 6.1. Psychologists' graduate training typically exposes them to various diagnostic techniques. The profession places high value on the techniques of uncovering and organizing psychosocial histories, as well as the proper choice, administration, and

EXHIBIT 6.1
Aspects of the Psychobiosocial Model Within the Diagnostic Phase

Psychologists use their unique skills to

1. differentiate problems along a continuum of function and dysfunction (e.g., situational stress vs. more severe psychological conditions);
2. differentiate psychological dysfunction from underlying medical conditions;
3. integrate evidenced-based research with individual psychobiosocial variables;
4. remain vigilant to changes in function and focus of treatment over time; and
5. frequently reassess progress through multimodal data gathering, including interviews, psychological measures, and relevant laboratory studies.

Psychologists thereby ensure that the medication targets the core of the disorder rather than mere symptoms.

interpretation of a broad range of assessment instruments that measure specific traits, symptomatology, and global functioning. In addition, psychologists are trained to interpret individual and group data. Thus, their education prepares them to practice, with judgment, in an evidenced-based manner. That psychologists can bring this broad range of assessment skills to the psychobiosocial model greatly enhances their effectiveness. The prescribing–medical psychologists who are ascribing to a psychobiosocial model are diligent in obtaining necessary laboratory tests as a part of the overall emphasis of ongoing assessment. Because prescribing–medical psychologists' diagnostic skills can be a major contribution to their effectiveness, medical–prescribing psychologists who are adopting the psychobiosocial model commit to very systematic data gathering, including the use of extensive interviews with patients and relevant collaterals and psychological measures of patient problems as well as their strengths. Furthermore, the prescribing–medical psychologists who are ascribing to the psychobiosocial model maintain ongoing monitoring of adherence to the agreed-on medication regime as well as emergence of any side effects, or new questions in regard to the treatment plan in general.

It is well accepted that our present diagnostic systems, the *Diagnostic and Statistical Manual of Mental Disorders* (4th ed., text rev.; American Psychiatric Association, 2000) and the International Classification of Diseases (ICD 9; World Health Organization, 2007), although helpful, are limited in many ways (e.g., Beutler & Malik, 2002). A critical analysis of these diagnostic systems is tangential to the substance of this chapter. Nevertheless, it is important to point out the categorical nature of these systems. Although qualifiers such as mild, moderate, acute, and chronic are attached to differentiate degrees of maladjustment, the model is intended to classify the individual into diagnostic groups.

In the traditional medical model, patients' symptoms are elicited, and diagnostic tests are administered so that a specific syndrome can be identified. Medications approved for treating that syndrome are then prescribed. In contrast, because of prescribing–medical psychologists' training in behavioral assessments and treatments, combined with their reliance on ongoing relationship building, the psychobiosocial paradigm is broadened to evaluate presenting problems along a continuum of resilience and vulnerability. At the time of this writing (see Chapter 8, this volume), prescribing–medical psychologists are not limited to, nor are they generally offering 15-min medication checks. As a result, there is greater opportunity to engage with their patients in-depth and to focus on complex behaviors that often fit more than one diagnostic category and change over time. This orientation is likely to have a salubrious effect on their approach to psychopharmacotherapy.

One implication of the ongoing reinterpretation of diagnoses is that prescribing–medical psychologists are sensitive to very mild forms of disorders. In these cases, although medication may help with the disorder, the prescribing–

medical psychologist who is adopting the psychobiosocial model will use psychological interventions first as the least invasive procedure. The consequence should and could be less prescribing of medications by prescribing–medical psychologists who are ascribing to a psychobiosocial model than by prescribers of other orientations. Indeed, observational data support this hypothesis (Wiggins & Cummings, 1998).

Another implication of prescribing–medical psychologists' broad understanding and application of diagnostic skills is their ability to select medications that address the nuances of a patient's complaints. The postdoctoral training in psychopharmacology for psychologists provides extensive background in this critical aspect of effective prescribing. Medical–prescribing psychologists can use their understanding of the effects of drugs on specific symptoms, symptom clusters, and brain circuits to select the medication most appropriate for the whole person within the context of their coping skills. For instance, a patient who complains of chronic insomnia and worry may benefit from a serotonergic agent working through the cortical–striatal–thalamic circuit, but he or she may also benefit from training in meditation and relaxation to gain greater autonomy in preparation for eventual tapering of the medication. It is important to clarify that the psychobiosocial model directs the prescribing–medical psychologist away from "chasing symptoms," in which medications are used to ease discomfort while deeper core concerns are ignored. The psychobiosocial approach is thorough, integrating an evaluation of underlying diagnoses with an understanding of the unique strengths and complexity of each patient.

A result of the emphasis on ongoing diagnosis in the psychobiosocial model is closer collaboration with physicians. It has always been incumbent on psychologists to identify underlying medical conditions and refer when appropriate. Prescribing–medical psychologists' advanced training in physiology, pathophysiology, and laboratory assessment, combined with their previously developed strength as diagnosticians, allows for increased effectiveness in identifying medical conditions. For example, in interviews of prescribing–medical psychologists (see Chapter 8, this volume), many psychologists mentioned that their ability to recognize when a patient is physically ill was greatly enhanced by their training in psychopharmacology. They reported much greater ability to discern medical conditions such as seizures, ulcers, cancer, hormonal disorders, and anemia.

Relationship-Building Phase

The psychobiosocial model considers the establishment of the therapeutic alliance central to therapeutic effectiveness. The importance of the therapeutic relationship cannot be overstated regardless of whether treatment involves psychotherapy, psychopharmacotherapy, or a combined approach.

The effect is so significant that it has been considered the best single predictor of psychotherapy outcome (Horvath & Symonds, 1991; Norcross, 2002). The impact is no less important during the implementation of psychopharmacotherapy. In fact, Krupnick et al. (1996) reported that the strength of the therapeutic relationship is a better predictor of outcome than the treatment method used, accounting for 21% of variance. This finding is not surprising because the power of placebo and the positive impact of an optimistic and hopeful attitude by the health care provider are well documented.

The prescribing–medical psychologist who uses the psychobiosocial model begins the process of relationship building with some guiding principles, as outlined in Exhibit 6.2. The first principle is that an educated patient is empowered to make the best decisions in regard to his or her treatment. Second, the decision to treat should start with the least invasive and longest lasting approach with the fewest side effects. This decision typically favors the use of psychotherapy over pharmacotherapy. At the same time, the prescribing–medical psychologist remains open to combined treatments when indicated. The decision is part science and part clinical judgment, because most patients seen in everyday clinical practice have more complicated profiles and circumstances than the specially selected participants included in randomized controlled trials (e.g., Seligman, 1995). Nevertheless, the psychobiosocial model posits that there are very few conditions (e.g., severe, recurrent depression; bipolar disorder; schizophrenia; other psychotic disorders) that require prompt use of psychotropics as an essential part of treatment.

It is important that the prescribing–medical psychologist maintains a certain level of circumspection in regard to the bias toward the preeminence

EXHIBIT 6.2
Aspects of the Psychobiosocial Model
Within the Relationship-Building Phase

Psychologists strengthen the relationship by considering patients' desires, which problems patients consider most distressful, and which side effects patients can tolerate.

Facilitating informed consent includes, but is not limited to, the following:

1. various drug effects;
2. time to therapeutic effect;
3. alternatives, indications–contraindications, side effects;
4. potential for dependence;
5. discontinuation issues;
6. drug interactions;
7. pros and cons of psychotherapy, medication, and both; and
8. patient-specific factors.

Psychologists foster the therapeutic alliance through close work with physicians, which enhances patients' sense of safety.

---

of psychotherapy and ensures that, through education, the patient receives a multifactoral explanation of the existing problem. The psychobiosocial model of prescribing presumes that the patient will maintain the locus of control in regard to treatment planning and will take on the lion's share of responsibility for behavior change. The psychobiosocial model does not circumscribe the nature of human suffering or problems with adaptation as a "chemical imbalance." Rather than imbuing psychotropics with the singular power to remit symptoms, these agents are considered but one of the many tools available, along with lifestyle and behavioral changes, to achieve relief. Because of this broad orientation, there is limited potential for overmedication and dependency on the doctor as the "giver of relief" or "healer."

Psychologists, by virtue of their training in psychotherapy that requires verbal exploration and nonpharmacologic techniques to effect behavior change, are well versed in the dynamics of relationship building. When a collaborative decision is made to add medications to the therapeutic encounter, the relationship can be affected by a number of additional variables, including the meaning patients ascribe to medication, the knowledge or misinformation they may have about certain medications, the patient's intellectual or linguistic capacity to understand the complexities of medication use, cultural and religious beliefs that pertain to medications and their side effects, and pressures to use or avoid use of medications. The prescribing–medical psychologist must incorporate these variables into both the informed consent and the ongoing dynamics of the therapeutic relationship. For instance, a patient may consider the introduction of the topic of medications as a sign of increased support or a validation of the severity of his or her illness (e.g., the patient may think, "My doctor wants to make sure I will get better faster," or "My doctor doesn't think I can work through this on my own," or "My doctor must think I'm really crazy"). Some patients may have no objections to medication but may be adamantly opposed to specific drugs within a class (e.g., "I would like something to help with depression, but not that Prozac . . . I hear it makes people homicidal"). Others may consider reliance on medication as a sign of spiritual weakness or lack of faith (e.g., "My minister says that if I just have enough faith and pray every day, God will help me overcome this depression"). The reasons for different reactions are as varied as the patients themselves, but the constancy of approach in attending to these factors is the common heuristic for the prescribing–medical psychologist. Therefore, informed consent is not only extensive, but it is used as a relationship-building tool throughout the therapy. Informed consent that is core to the psychobiosocial model includes educating as well as listening to patients' responses in an effort to strengthen the potential for adherence to the treatment plan and positive therapeutic outcome.

Of course, the psychobiosocial model incorporates the standards of practice in regard to informed consent that other medical managers use, including information about risks, benefits, alternatives, and side effects of various medications. However, as noted earlier, patient-specific factors, such as the impact a particular medication may have on the individual's weight, lipid and insulin levels, blood pressure, sexual performance, or irritability, may have specific meaning to patients, depending on their medical status, level of anxiety or dysmorphophobia, or relationship dynamics with their marital partner or significant other. The prescribing–medical psychologist would include these factors when tailoring pharmacotherapeutic suggestions to the patient's needs, desires, goals, or concerns. For instance, a patient may have minimal risk factors for metabolic syndrome but have a significant family history of cardiovascular disease and fear of weight gain. In this case, using a medication that is likely to increase triglycerides, weight, or blood pressure may result in greater risk than benefit based on the patient's history and anxieties. If alternatives with fewer metabolic side effects are available, these should be considered, and an explanation as to why the patient might choose one over another should be offered when decisions concerning choice of a medication are made.

As another example, an anorexic patient who is purposely losing weight because of dysmorphophobia should be informed of the potential for weight gain with use of specific psychotropics rather than surreptitiously using the weight gain side effect as a therapeutic intervention. Further, a patient who is attempting to salvage a marriage may consider the potential sexual dysfunction with selective serotonin reuptake inhibitors (SSRIs) to outweigh the potential benefits. Such is the case of a 47-year-old woman who was experiencing marital discord and was threatened with separation by her husband because of problems with patient's increased irritability and decreased libido. According to the patient, her husband equated lack of love making with a lack of love in the relationship. The introduction of an SSRI, such as paroxetine, with the potential for delayed orgasm or anorgasmia that could compound the decreased libido, would likely exacerbate the existing relationship dynamics and outweigh the benefit to depressive irritability. These efforts to tailor the risks, benefits, and alternatives not only to the medical but also the psychological and social effects of the medication are more likely to increase the trust in the therapist and, by extension, enhance the therapeutic relationship, the likelihood of medication adherence, and the therapeutic benefit of the medication.

Interactions between the patient's existing regimen and potential new agents should be explained and considered as well. These interactions are not always considered negative by the patient; and, again, explanations should be tailored to the specific patient. For instance, adding a medication that has an additive anorexic effect for a patient who is taking an appetite suppressant may be a welcome addition for some patients. Similarly, adding a medicine with sedative properties to the nighttime regimen of an individual who is already taking a hypnotic without full resolution of insomnia may be considered a welcome interaction as long as there are no other significant untoward side effects.

Another important characteristic of the psychobiosocial model is that the psychologist acts as a consultant rather than as a medical authority who issues orders based on the prescriber's knowledge and expertise. There are times when a patient will demand, "You are the doctor; you are supposed to tell me what to take." In these cases, as with so many that require active listening and interpretation, the patient's response should be considered within the context of the therapeutic relationship. For instance, is the patient jokingly marveling at the newfound opportunity to make his own medical decisions? Is the patient dependent in personality style and feeling uncomfortable about making independent decisions? Is the patient suffering from anxiety and subsequent ambivalence about making the wrong choice? Exploration of these questions with the patient is fodder for strengthening the therapeutic relationship and can serve to enhance psycho- and pharmacotherapeutic benefits. It is important to note that a patient's needs, desires, goals, and concerns in addition to their medication regimen can and do change from session to session. Therefore, it is important to ensure that the relationship building remains active and dynamic with each interaction.

An important aspect of the relationship-building phase that invariably begins at the time of initial assessment is the expectation of collaboration between the prescribing–medical psychologist and the patient's primary care physician. This relationship has become increasingly important with the recognition of many adverse physical effects catalyzed by psychotropic intervention. The metabolic syndrome that can be precipitated by antipsychotics, particularly the newer ones, always warrants close monitoring. Other possibilities to be considered include syndrome of inappropriate diuretic hormone, toxic epidermal necrolysis, agranulocytosis, and thrombocytopenia, all of which can be caused by various psychotropics. In addition, prescribing–medical psychologists should ensure that treatment of the mental health patient incorporates principles of physical health and health monitoring into the treatment planning. The collaboration between the patients' psychologist and primary care doctor not only informs the patient that these data are necessary and valuable but also offers a potent message to patients that they are valuable and worthy of the doctors' making contact on their behalf.

Active-Working Phase

In general, the active-working phase is characterized by in vivo change. The relationship between patients and their therapists may be used within the therapeutic session as a method of enhancing the adaptive process and to help patients to better understand their perceptions and reaction to others. Psychologists work to educate patients about their problems, not only as a constellation of symptoms belonging to broader diagnosis but also as part of a continuum of adaptation and maladaptation, function and dysfunction. The goal is to avoid a reductionistic model that distills symptoms to a singular disease in favor of a more holistic and integrative approach. The patients' problems are viewed within the context of systems and overall integrity of function, teaching new skills and behaviors in response to stress. The psychologist often uses the strength of the therapeutic rapport to instill hope and reinforce constructive–adaptive behaviors. Exhibit 6.3 outlines some major aspects of the active-working phase.

In a traditional medical model, medication compliance is interpreted behaviorally as a willingness to follow or not follow the prescriber's specific recommendations. In the prescribing–medical psychologist's psychobiosocial model of care, medication adherence is considered one more way to understand the patient's psychological functioning. The patient's attitudes toward and reactions to the medication are viewed in the context of the interpersonal event. In psychodynamic terms, the medication can be viewed as a transference object. For example, if a patient is very anxious, it is not unlikely

EXHIBIT 6.3
Aspects of the Psychobiosocial Model Within the Active-Working Phase

Work of the early phases continues.

Psychologists use medication as a tool of intra- and interpersonal change.

Medication selection and use—understood within the context of personal meaning to the patient—increase adherence and facilitate change.

Psychologists collaborate extensively with patients about medication effects and side effects. This collaboration can do the following:

1. increase the patients' sense of autonomy;
2. increase adherence; and
3. lead to more effective education and confrontation when drug-seeking behaviors are observed to assist with alternative treatments and coping strategies, especially among substance abusers and those with chronic pain.

Psychologists analyze suboptimal or diminished effects of medications within the context of pharmacokinetics and pharmacodynamics, as well as evaluate new stressors; secondary gains; unrealistic expectations; placebo effect; and increasing awareness of psychological, physical, and social impacts.

Psychologists' techniques of reframing and supporting an internal locus of control help patients "own the success" of the intervention, thereby building patient confidence and autonomy.

that he or she will be apprehensive about taking medication; further, the patient may be hypervigilant to bodily changes or mild side effects from the medication. These reactions can be clinically significant, particularly in those patients with panic disorder. In the psychologist's psychobiosocial model of care, this response is not ignored but is carefully considered in the therapy session. Whether one is approaching the matter psychodynamically through interpretation or through behavioral and cognitive analysis, the patient's hesitancy about the medication because of an underlying anxiety can be discussed as an example of how his or her anxiety prevents optimal functioning. In a similar fashion, a patient's refusal to follow instructions in taking medication despite a collaborative decision to initiate such treatment may be an indication of some fear, unexpressed concerns, acting out, or antisocial tendencies. In such cases, the psychologist will help the patient analyze whether the lack of appropriate follow through is part of a greater pattern of difficulty. For example, when issues of trust or power impact compliance, these are discussed in therapy so that the patient learns how these attitudes can prevent optimal functioning in the therapy session as well as in other environments. When the lack of follow through springs from other difficulties, such as cognitive deficits, discomfort with side effects, unexpressed concerns, or social or other pressures, these are also fully explored.

Within the active-working phase, psychotropics can be used as a tool for increasing patient autonomy. Psychologists are concerned not only with ameliorating patient symptoms but also with maximizing patients' growth and resilience. As a consequence, educating patients about themselves and their environments and offering them extensive informed consent about medications are central to the psychologist's practice. Along with learning about the psychosocial environment, the patient also learns about the medications, their effects, and side effects in a first-hand and experiential manner within the active-working phase. Using the psychotropic as a tool for building autonomy can be particularly useful for patients with low self-esteem, problematic dependency needs, or both. As therapy continues, the psychologist increasingly asks and defers to the patient's informed judgment about the medications. Initially, insecure patients may respond, "I don't know. You're the doctor." However, as the psychologist continues to entrust the decision making to the patient, the psychologist's belief in the patient's competence instills greater self-esteem. Using the medication as a tool for building healthy autonomy may be useful for patients with other difficulties.

During this active-working phase, psychologists use psychological techniques of reframing toward the goal of patients who are integrating an internal locus of control about their enhanced functioning. In traditional psychotropic medication management, patients often finish treatment with a sense that their gains are primarily dependent on the effects of the medication. Certainly, the fact that mental illness is often presented to these patients as strictly a biological event, a chemical imbalance, reinforces this perception. In addition, however, the medication manager may not have the time or the theoretical orientation to highlight the specific changes the patient has made in his or her cognitions or behaviors. The prescribing–medical psychologist who is adopting the psychobiosocial model rigorously emphasizes to patients that the medications help them reach sufficient equanimity so that they can access their own strengths and enact fundamental, self-directed changes in their lives. An internal locus of control can enhance self-esteem and encourage proactive behavior (Rotter, 1990). Therefore, reframing the medication effect as part of the patient's overall change for which the patient should take credit is a way of strengthening the patient's ego, imbuing the patient with hope for the future, and fostering goal setting and assertive behaviors to reach those goals.

Another aspect and benefit of the psychologist's psychobiosocial model of care that is strongly evidenced in the active-working phase is a result of the extensive informed consent that involves collaboration and agreement by the patient and psychologist. In traditional medical management of mental disorders, when a patient experiences untoward effects, the prescriber often makes a unilateral decision about how to change the medication. In contrast, the prescribing–medical psychologist educates the patient in an ongoing way about side effects and drug interactions. Sharpening the patient's skills of self-observation is an effective component of psychotherapy. In the psychobiosocial model of care used by the prescribing–medical psychologist, patients increase their insight into the effects of their behavior and effects of the medications that they take. Therefore, they develop increasing psychological and medical mindedness that can be of significant usefulness in their lives. This increase in psychological and medical mindedness leads naturally into the generalization phase.

Generalization Phase

Within the generalization phase, outlined in Exhibit 6.4, patients transfer learning from the therapeutic session to their everyday lives. In the active-working phase patients learned a great deal about themselves and their medication. They have learned about the biological, psychological, and social correlates of their distress; and they have accrued a basic understanding of how the medications work, in general, and how they work in their lives, specifically. For instance, patients have developed rudimentary skills in analyzing the personal effects and side effects of medications and the costs and benefits associated with their use. Then, during the generalization phase, patients increasingly apply this learning. For example, they may initiate discussions of whether or not a medication is still working effectively, or they

EXHIBIT 6.4
Aspects of the Psychobiosocial Model Within the Generalization Phase

Patients actively seek opportunities to transfer learning to old and new situations, approaching past difficulties with greater equanimity and venturing into challenging situations with new behaviors.

Patients learn to become expert observers of themselves and understand the need for psychotherapy, medication, or both.

Patients learn to monitor and balance the dynamic and reciprocal interaction between life circumstances and medication effects. As a result, they can do the following:

1. cope with long-term side effects if necessary;
2. identify and enact desired changes in the psychosocial environment prompted by personal growth; and
3. recognize when certain side effects are no longer tolerable because of changes in the psychosocial environment.

Patients assume increasing responsibility for the enhancement of their well-being, including identifying symptoms, side effects, and the need to change.

may become aware that there are new issues of central concern that should be addressed either in the therapy, with psychotropics, or both. In other words, they develop expertise in observing themselves, both in terms of their psychological functioning and their need for medication. As the patient develops these skills, the prescribing–medical psychologist is respectful of his or her ideas and points out the patient's increased skill at self-observation. Reinforcing the patient's skill at self-observation becomes another tool for increasing sense of autonomy. Self-esteem is enhanced when patients feel more capable of identifying their needs and alternative ways to change.

With the addition of psychotropic intervention, there is greater opportunity for incorporating the newly experienced somatic and kinesthetic states with new insights and behaviors. An illustrative example of how these states can be incorporated into the patient's daily life is evidenced in the case of Mr. Jones, a 34-year-old man who was experiencing anxiety. For several days before a planned social event or a deadline at work, he would ruminate about a myriad of negative outcomes. During the days leading up to the event, he would feel increased muscle tension, headaches, and irritability and was worried that he could lash out at any moment, if stressed. His prescribing–medical psychologist initially attempted to use behavioral techniques for anxiety management, and he showed some success with these techniques. However, he continued to feel overwhelmed by his worry and irritability. He was treated with an SSRI, and after 6 weeks, he began to describe greater control over his worry and less irritability with greater patience. He described the changes in somatic sensations: "I just don't get that big knot in my stomach . . . that pressure in my chest that I normally get when I feel like exploding." He went on to describe that the tension and subsequent compulsion to act in violent or verbally aggressive ways had dissipated. Mr. Jones was encouraged to seek out situations he found anxiety provoking or irritating and to specifically focus on the sensations of calm in that moment while using self-soothing, affirming statements. In this way, he could take advantage of the anxiety dampening associated with the SSRI while establishing new adaptive, autonomous behaviors. Connecting with the sensations of calm rather than the usual experience of autonomic hyperarousal was a new experience for him, and the therapy allowed him to associate the physical sensation with his developing identity as someone who was no longer controlled by his emotional or physical state. He was reminded to use relaxation procedures as another skill to promote similar somatic and kinesthetic experiences.

This illustration is useful for demonstrating many of the principles inherent to the generalization phase insofar as the patient is learning to become an expert observer of his thoughts, feelings and physical states. It demonstrates another critical component of the psychobiosocial model in that it shows how the patient is encouraged to assume increasing responsibility for the enhancement of his own well being rather than assuming a fatalistic and dependent view of the effect of the medication.

There may be occasions when the medication does not alleviate as much of the anxiety as Mr. Jones or other patients may wish, and these represent fertile opportunities for the prescribing–medical psychologist to encourage use of behavioral techniques such as deep abdominal breathing, autogenic–progressive muscle relaxation, mindfulness, or worry scheduling during those stressful times. Combining these therapeutic techniques with the psychotropic intervention assists the patient in maintaining the greatest degree of autonomy while transferring new learning to familiar and novel situations, thereby promoting resilience and personal growth. This greater sense of achievement and self-reliance enhances the patient's ability to identify and enact desired changes in the psychosocial environment.

As they become expert observers and self-supporters, patients consider the need for continued medication and begin to reconsider the question, "How long am I supposed to stay on this stuff?" Such questions are often a signal to the therapist that the dynamic process of self-awareness, goal setting, and perhaps improved functioning with concomitant thoughts of termination are prompting the patient to review the long-term benefits and risks of medication. It may also be that their social environment has changed. For example, the divorcee who was able to tolerate sexual side effects when compared with suicidal thoughts over the intense grief and depression associated with losing his marriage may reunite with his spouse, and, consequently, feel that the sexual dysfunction is too great a cost in this phase of his life. The generalization phase is predicated on the concept of patient as capable of change that can extend to all spheres of life. When these changes have been implemented successfully or with significant progress, it is common to consider the termination phase of treatment.

Termination Phase

Psychologists well understand the importance of terminating therapy in a sensitive fashion. If issues of anxiety and attachment are not carefully addressed within this phase, many of the patient's gains can be compromised. A prescribing–medical psychologist who adopts the psychobiosocial model of care understands the importance of discussing in detail aspects of termination of the relationship and also possible termination of medication, and critical aspects of the termination process in the psychobiosocial model are identified in Exhibit 6.5. Because the prescribing–medical psychologist has addressed the issue of locus of control in the active-working phase, some of the difficulties encountered in traditional psychotropic medication management may be obviated. For instance, patients may feel perfectly capable and primed for determining when progress is sufficiently advanced and stable enough to consider discontinuation of psychopharmacotherapy, or they may realize that their use of medications will be a life-long commitment.

Despite the preparatory work of the active and generalization phases, certain patients struggle with terminating medication. As in psychotherapy, some want to terminate prematurely, whereas others have difficulty letting go of the assistance. In some cases, patients may wish to hold on to the medication as a connection to the security provided by the therapy regardless of a lack of empirical support for long-term use. In psychodynamic terms, the medication can be viewed in these cases as a transitional object in which patients imbue the medication with a facility to create the positive feelings associated

EXHIBIT 6.5
Aspects of the Psychobiosocial Model During the Termination Phase

The psychologist assesses whether and how rapidly the psychotherapy and pharmacotherapy should be terminated.

If the patient progresses to maintenance sessions, the psychologist discusses the change in frequency and content of therapy, as well as qualitative changes in the therapeutic relationship.

The patient deals with fears about stopping psychotherapy or stopping the pharmacotherapy (which may include reviewing attachment issues and over-reliance on pharmacological interventions).

with the therapist and therapeutic process. An appropriate response for such cases is to refocus patients on the internal changes in their mood and increased adaptation so that they are more confident about their changes and personal growth. In addition to knowledge of psychopharmacology and awareness of biopsychosocial factors likely to influence functioning once medications are discontinued, prescribing–medical psychologists use a variety of clinical skills such as active listening, observation, interpretation, reinforcement, and education to help patients to determine the appropriateness of and their readiness to discontinue psychopharmacotherapy.

Of course, patients with chronic difficulties may require long-term psychotropic intervention. In the psychologist's psychobiosocial model of care, follow-up sessions, although less frequent and of shorter duration than during the active treatment, still include psychotherapy and psychosocial interventions, as well as medication management components. Very often, during traditional maintenance of psychotropic medications, the practitioner checks on symptoms and lowers or increases medications accordingly. In addition, the prescribing–medical psychologist continues to query about the level of functioning and psychosocial stressors. If there is reason to suspect a worsening of the condition or of current stressors, more frequent sessions may be reinitiated and medication may be titrated, or the patient may be reminded of the potential value that results from continued adherence. In this way, maintenance sessions become opportunities not only to sustain the gains already established in treatment but to also proactively avoid impediments to optimal functioning.

It is important to note that adoption of the psychobiosocial model in the long-term maintenance with serious mental illness is congruent with current thinking that the goal for this population should be "recovery." As explained in the President's New Freedom Commission on Mental Health report (2003):

> (1) the [present] system is not oriented to the single most important goal of the people it serves—the hope of recovery; (2) "the system should foster recovery, resilience, and independence; and (3) Research and personal testimony confirm that "recovery from mental illness is real: there are a range of effective treatments, services, and supports to the facilitate recovery. (p. 76)

By continuing to work with these patients to increase self-efficacy and self-determination and to change personal narratives (Lysaker, Lancaster, & Lysaker, 2003; Roe, 2003) as well as to monitor medication effects and side effects, patients continue to grow over time and are more likely to reach recovery. The prescribing–medical psychologist's active-working stance continues throughout the maintenance phase until the patient is able to achieve "a satisfying, hopeful, and contributing life even with limitations caused by the illness" (Anthony, 1993, p. 11).

Last, when treating long-term cases and moving into a maintenance phase, the prescribing–medical psychologist who is adopting a psychobiosocial model does not assume that the patient understands that the relationship changes after termination of regular sessions but rather carefully explains the change in the relationship. During the termination phase and in maintenance sessions, the psychologist inquires how the patient is dealing with this relationship change.

APPLICATION OF THE MODEL TO SEVERAL CRITICAL MENTAL HEALTH ISSUES

Individuals With Severe Mental Illness

Presently, adults with serious mental illness treated in public systems die an average of 25 years earlier than Americans overall. In the 1990s, those with mental illness tended to die 10 to 15 years earlier. Thus, the mortality gap between the mentally ill and other Americans has widened significantly in the last 20 years. The high-mortality incidence among the mentally ill is related, in part, to higher accident and suicide rates. However, three out of five mentally ill persons died from preventable diseases (Colton & Manderscheid, 2006; Daly, 2008). Many of the treatable diseases are associated with metabolic syndrome characterized by hypertension, insulin resistance or glucose intolerance, and hypercholesteremia. Prevalence studies reveal a two- to four-fold increased risk of metabolic syndrome among patients with schizophrenia compared with demographically matched peers (Meyer, 2007). Lifestyle and personal habits such as poor nutrition and higher smoking rates contribute to this extremely serious condition. It is also known that a number of the atypical antipsychotics as well as the traditional antipsychotics increase the risk of metabolic syndrome. Application of the psychobiosocial model presented within this chapter suggests multiple means for potentially reducing the mortality rate among individuals who are suffering from severe mental illness.

Within the Diagnostic Phase

The psychobiosocial model suggests that prescribing–medical psychologists will need to address issues of limited self-care and lack of social support that are common among individuals with severe mental illness. This aspect of care had already received attention clinically and through research by psychologists prior to the advancement of prescriptive authority. In addition, the model calls for careful, frequent, and holistic monitoring of overall functioning to include maladaptive behaviors such as smoking, use of alcohol and illicit substances, and poor dietary habits. The psychobiosocial model implies reliance on a multidisciplinary approach to treatment, with increased referral to other health professionals when it is believed that biological factors are affecting or are likely to affect functioning. Because prescribing–medical psychologists who are working under the psychobiosocial model meet with their patients often, side effects are frequently monitored and addressed in a timely fashion. As patients demonstrate signs of improvement and sustained, stable functioning, the psychopharmacotherapeutic regimen may be altered or reduced with augmentation through consistent psychological and social strategies.

Within the Relationship-Building Phase

Prescribing–medical psychologists recognize that all patients, including individuals with severe mental illness, can become educated consumers of services. Through the collaborative relationship with the psychologist, patients learn the best way to manage their difficulties. The close relationship with the patient enhances compliance to recommendations in regard to diet, medication, and stressors. Greater reliance on the therapeutic alliance and psychosocial interventions may have the net effect of minimizing the need for multiple, redundant medications, potentially decreasing the likelihood of metabolic syndrome and other serious side effects. In the relationship-building phase, the prescribing–medical psychologist who ascribes to a psychobiosocial model serves as an important liaison with other treating individuals for these vulnerable patients. Because of the ongoing multidisciplinary relationship with the primary care physician and other professionals, the fragmentation of services so characteristic for this vulnerable population can be minimized, leading to more effective and safer overall care.

Within the Active-Working Phase

In addition to the biologically based symptoms, patients with severe mental illness often develop feelings of helplessness and hopelessness because of the strict controls within long-term institutional settings and the fragmentation of care in outpatient settings. In the psychobiosocial model, the prescribing–medical psychologist integrates education as well as psychotherapeutic techniques to build a sense of autonomy. Hence, patients are taught coping, self-soothing, and problem-solving skills to enhance self-sufficiency. With increased awareness and sense of autonomy, some patients may be more likely to address habits such as smoking that are associated with their higher rate of mortality. In addition, as a part of the active-working phase, the prescribing–medical psychologist helps the patient with severe mental illness to address negative symptoms of psychosis with psychotherapy as well as medication.

Because patients learn to be more effective personally and socially, they can build a stronger network of support. The quality of their life and daily self-care can improve accordingly. As mentioned previously, an emerging body of literature substantiates that with sufficient psychological as well as medication intervention, those with severe mental illness can become functional and that the quality of their physical and personal lives does improve. The prescribing–medical psychologist who adopts a psychobiosocial model is particularly equipped to achieve these promising goals.

Within the Generalization Phase

As the prescribing–medical psychologist helps the severely mentally ill develop social networks, these networks can buffer against relapse. Care becomes more proactive, avoiding increased medications and hospitalizations associated with severe relapse and concomitant medical and financial side effects. Also, because the prescribing–medical psychologist who uses a psychobiosocial model maintains a close relationship with the patient through the working and generalization phases, there is less likelihood of patients using medications inconsistently. Thus, the reduction in benefit that can result when a medication is reintroduced is minimized, which in turn can contribute to using lower levels of medication (Carlat, 2008). Those with severe mental illness who are treated by the prescribing–medical psychologist who uses the psychobiosocial model of care will retain their increased psychological and medication mindedness and sense of autonomy through the generalization phase, further decreasing their learned helplessness and sense of hopelessness. As their worlds broaden, they are able to seek services and further improve their lifestyles so that they are healthier, psychologically and medically.

Within the Termination Phase

Within the prescribing–medical psychologist's psychobiosocial model of care, severely mentally ill persons are maintained in a long-term psychotherapeutic–medication management relationship with the provider. In follow-up sessions, patients continue to learn new coping mechanisms, and stressors that could trigger relapse are noted and addressed. These periodic medication and psychotherapy checks serve as prophylaxis against future illness episodes, thereby decreasing the risk of suicide, accidents, and unhealthy side effects that are due to higher medication levels.

Antidepressant Black Box Warnings

The Food and Drug Administration (FDA) black box warnings, placed on antidepressant labels, in regard to suicidality with the use of antidepressants state,

Antidepressants increase the risk compared to placebo of suicidal thinking and behavior (suicidality) in children, adolescents, and young adults in short-term studies of major depressive disorders (MDD) and other psychiatric disorders. Anyone considering the use of Fluoxetine or any other antidepressant in a child, adolescent or young adult must balance this risk with the clinical need. Short-term studies did not show an increase in the risk of suicidality with the use of antidepressants compared to placebo in adults beyond age 24; there was a reduction in risk with antidepressants compared to placebo in adults aged 65 and older. (Physicians' Desk Reference, 2010, p. 1941)

This warning defines suicidality as "a heightened risk of suicidal thinking and behavior." According to FDA data, none of the children in the experimental group actually committed suicide despite the higher incidence of suicidal thinking.

Although the warning has been very important in reducing the liberal use of antidepressants, there is evidence that in some cases the black box warning may be adversely changing clinical practice patterns. According to Cordero, Rudd, Bryan, and Corso (2008), over 90% of those primary care doctors interviewed believe the black box warning referred to an increased risk of death rather than suicidal thinking and behavior. As a consequence, these physicians were less willing to prescribe psychotropics and were also more reluctant to refer for psychotropic treatment (Gibbons et al., 2007; Lineberry et al., 2007). Most distressing is the possibility that adding the black box warning in 2004 has actually resulted in an increase in completed suicides among children and adolescents (Gibbons et al., 2007).

Within the Diagnostic Phase

The prescribing–medical psychologist is quite skilled in differentiating disorders such as grief and transient situational stress from clinical depression and will begin with the least invasive, nonpsychotropic interventions whenever appropriate. Similarly, the prescribing–medical psychologist is trained to recognize medical disorders that may mask the psychological conditions and to refer those cases to physicians rather than to treat with antidepressants. Thus, prescribing–medical psychologists who use the psychobiosocial model are likely to use antidepressants with a more select child and adolescent population. On the other hand, if the use of an antidepressant is warranted, the prescribing–medical psychologist is trained in research methodology to explain the warning accurately. Furthermore, because of the close relationship with the patient, the prescribing–medical psychologist will monitor the suicidal thinking frequently and judiciously.

Within the Relationship Building Phase

Prescribing–medical psychologists enhance the safety net because patients are actively engaged in monitoring their reactions, including their suicidal thinking. Further, when prescribing–medical psychologists use a psychobiosocial model, the family is actively engaged in monitoring for suicidal thinking and behavior. The family's fears can be further allayed when the prescribing–medical psychologist collaborates with the PCP so that the patient knows that there are multiple sources of support with whom to consult about any untoward reactions.

Within the Active Working Phase

During this phase, any lack of follow-through of the agreed-on psychotropic regimen will be identified and discussed with the patient in relationship to the patient's personal fears and trust in the therapeutic relationship. As a consequence, the therapeutic relationship is enhanced, and the psychologist is more assured that the patient will report suicidal thinking and behavior. Also, the prescribing–medical psychologist's trust in the competence of the patient and the family creates a team orientation, further enhancing the patient's autonomy. As the patient's self-reliance increases, the patient is less likely to be swayed impulsively by suicidal thinking, and more likely to report such thoughts to others. Discussion of the risk of increased suicidal ideation becomes an excellent opportunity to increase the patient's psychological and medical mindedness. The extensive informed consent about increased suicidality increases the young patient's sense of responsibility of self and thus enhances an internal locus of control for his or her successful changes.

Within the Generalization Phase

In this phase, patients transfer learning about the side effects of the antidepressants to their understanding of other psychological symptoms and use of other medications. Thus, even child and adolescent patients learn to make wiser choices about interventions in the future. Because patients learn about the seriousness of using these medications, both potential benefits and side effects, the patients are better equipped to ascertain when it is appropriate to stop the antidepressant or other medication, and they are less likely to stop medication prematurely. It is even possible that the learning could transfer to a more judicious consideration of the use of over-the-counter or street drugs. Thus, by actively addressing the black box warning about antidepressants, these young patients can become better educated consumers of all chemical substances as well as their mental health treatment.

Within the Termination Phase

Because the issue is used to enhance young patients' sense of responsibility for their own care, follow-through in the termination phase can be improved. Furthermore, patients will be able to evaluate their needs for antidepressant medication more objectively in the future.

CONCLUSION

The causes of the worldwide crisis in mental health care and the breakdown in the mental health care system in the United States in particular are complex and multiple. Clearly, the dearth of sufficient providers, as well as the limitations in training that create fragmented care, are important contributors. Prescribing–medical psychologists, adopting the psychobiosocial model of care, can be an important part of the solution to this crisis. An integrated psychobiosocial model of care, including cognitive and behavioral intervention, changes in the social environment, and psychotropic aid, is often more efficacious in patient treatment, especially complex cases. Prescribing–medical psychologists are well trained to integrate these interventions into a psychobiosocial model because they have completed specialized postdoctoral training programs. The prescribing–medical psychologists are experienced in critically analyzing pharmaceutical studies so that the prescribing practices are empirically based. The prescribing–medical psychologists' extensive history taking and objective measures facilitate the evaluation of client gain as well as drug efficacy. Thus, the medication used in conjunction with psychological and behavioral intervention can provide maximum care with limited side effects. It is important to note that the power to prescribe is also the power to unprescribe and limit untoward effects. In present-day practice, biological and social interventions are often not well integrated. Prescribing–medical psychologists' close collaboration with primary care physicians provides more thorough medical care and more holistic care. Extensive collaboration with patients about medication effects and side effects (i.e., broad informed consent in the tradition of "giving psychology away"; Miller, 1969) increases compliance and patient autonomy.

In this chapter, we have attempted to present the skeleton of a prescribing–medical psychologist psychobiosocial model in a manner that will encourage further critical thinking. Although the model is incomplete and based on some speculation, we hope that it will prompt further specification and elaboration as well as critical analysis and refinements. In his *Interpretation of Dreams*, Freud (1900/1998) wisely provided the following caveat to his postulates:

I see no necessity to apologize for the imperfections of this or any similar imagery. Analogies of this kind are only intended to assist us in our attempt to make the complications of mental functioning intelligible by dissecting the function and assigning the different constituents to different component parts of the apparatus. . . . We are justified, in my view, in giving free rein to our speculations as long as we retain the coolness of our judgment and do not mistake the scaffolding for the building. (p. 575)

We hope that the ideas presented in this chapter can prompt development of a model of critical functionality that can be used to replicate the psychobiosocial treatment approach and, eventually, can serve to test the efficacy of the model against other approaches. This will help create an effective shelter to address the global crisis in mental health care.

REFERENCES

American Psychiatric Association. (2000). *Diagnostic and statistical manual of mental disorders* (4th ed., text rev.). Washington, DC: Author.

Anthony, W. A. (1993). Recovering from mental illness: The guiding vision of the mental health service system in the 1990's. *Psychosocial Rehabilitation Journal, 16,* 11–23.

Beutler, L. E., & Malik, M. L. (Eds.). (2002). *Rethinking the DSM: A psychological perspective.* Washington, DC: American Psychological Association. doi:10.1037/10456-000

Carlat, D. (2008, February). The kindling hypothesis: It is relevant to psychiatry? *Carlat Psychiatry Report, 6*(2). Retrieved from http://www.thecarlatreport.com/article/kindling-hypothesis-it-relevant-psychiatry

Cordero, L., Rudd, M., Bryan, C., & Corso, K. (2008). Accuracy of primary care medical providers' understanding of the FDA black box warning label for antidepressants. *Primary Care & Community Psychiatry, 13,* 109–114.

Colton, C. W., & Manderscheid, R. W. (2006). Congruencies in increased mortality rates, years of potential life lost, and causes of death among public mental health clients in eight states. *Preventing Chronic Disease, 3,* A42. Retrieved from http://www.cdc.gov/pcd/issues/2006/apr/05_0180.htm.

Daly, R. (2008). Untreated chronic illness blamed for high mortality. *Psychiatric News, 43,* 7.

de Jonghe, F., Kool, S., van Aalst, J., Dekker, J., & Peen, J. (2001). Combining psychotherapy and antidepressants in the treatment of depression. *Journal of Affective Disorders, 64,* 217–229.

Engel, G. L. (1977, April 8). The need for a new medical model: A challenge for biomedicine. *Science, 196,* 129–136. doi:10.1126/science.847460

Freud, S. (1998). *The interpretation of dreams*. New York, NY: Basic Books. (Original work published 1900)

Gibbons, R. D., Brown, C. H., Hur, K., Marcus, S. M., Bhaumik, D. K., Erkins, J. A., . . . Mann, J. J. (2007). Early evidence on the effects of regulators' suicidality warnings on SSRI prescriptions and suicide in children and adolescents. *The American Journal of Psychiatry, 164,* 1356–1363. doi:10.1176/appi.ajp.2007.07030454

Goodwin, F. K., & Jamison, K. R. (2007). *Manic depressive illness: Bipolar disorders and recurrent depression*. Oxford, England: Oxford University Press.

Hogarty, G. E. (1993). Prevention of relapse in chronic schizophrenic patients. *The Journal of Clinical Psychiatry, 54*(Suppl), 18–23.

Hollon, S. D. (1996). The efficacy and effectiveness of psychotherapy relative to medications. *American Psychologist, 51,* 1025–1030.

Hollon, S. D., Jarrett, R. B., Nieremberg, A. A., Thase, M. E., Trivedi, M., & Rush, A. J. (2005). Psychotherapy and medication in the treatment of adult and geriatric depression: Which monotherapy or combined treatment? *The Journal of Clinical Psychiatry, 66,* 455–468.

Horvath, A. O., & Symonds, B. D. (1991). Relation between working alliance and outcome in psychotherapy: A meta-analysis. *Journal of Counseling Psychology, 38,* 139–149. doi:10.1037/0022-0167.38.2.139

Jensen, P., Arnold, E., Swanson, J., Vitiello, B., Abikoff, H., Greenhill, L., et al. (2007). Three-year follow-up of the NIMH MTA study. *Journal of the American Academy of Child and Adolescent Psychology, 46,* 989–1002. doi:10.1097/CHI.0b013e3180686d48

Kennard, B. D., Silva, S., Vitiello, B., Curry, J., & Kratochvil, C. (2009). Readmission and residual symptoms after acute treatment of adolescents with major depressive disorder. *Journal of the American Academy of Child and Adolescent Psychiatry, 48,* 186–195. doi:10.1097/CHI.0b013e31819176f9

Krupnick, J. L., Sotsky, S. M., Simmens, S., Moyer, J., Elkin, I., Watkins, J., & Pilkonis, P. A. (1996). The role of therapeutic alliance in psychotherapy and pharmacotherapy outcome: Findings in the National Institute of Mental Health Treatment of Depression Collaborative Research Program. *Journal of Clinical Psychology, 64,* 532–539.

Leichsenring, F., & Rabung, S. (2008). Effectiveness of long-term psychodynamic psychotherapy: A meta-analysis. *JAMA, 300,* 1551–1565. doi:10.1001/jama.300.13.1551

Lineberry, T. W., Botswick, J. M., Beebe, T. J., & Decker, P. A. (2007). Impact of the FDA black box warning on physician antidepressant prescribing practice patterns: Opening Pandora's suicide box. *Mayo Clinic Proceedings, 82,* 518–520. doi:10.4065/82.4.518

Lysaker, P. H., Lancaster, R. S., & Lysaker, J. T. (2003). Narrative transformation as an outcome in the psychotherapy of schizophrenia. *Psychology and Psychotherapy: Theory, Research and Practice, 76,* 285–299. doi:10.1348/147608303322362505

Meyer, J. M. (2007). The metabolic syndrome and schizophrenia: Clinical research update. *Psychiatric Times*, *24*, 1–2. Retrieved from http://www.psychiatrictimes.com/schizophrenia/article/10168/46441pagenumbers=2

Miller, G. A. (1969). Psychology as a means of promoting human welfare. *American Psychologist*, *24*, 1063–1075. doi:10.1037/h0028988

Norcross, J. C. (Ed.). (2002). *Psychotherapy relationships that work: Therapist contributions and responsiveness to patients*. New York, NY: Oxford University Press.

Olfson, M., & Marcus, S. (2009). National patterns in antidepressant medication treatment. *Archives of General Psychiatry*, *66*, 848–856. doi:10.1001/archgenpsychiatry.2009.81

Pampallona, S., Bollini, P., & Tibaldi, G. (2004). Combined pharmacotherapy and psychological treatment for depression. *Archives of General Psychiatry*, *61*, 714–719. doi:10.1001/archpsyc.61.7.714

Perlick, D. A., Rosenheck, R. A., Clarkin, J. F., Sirey, J., & Raue, P. (1999). Symptoms predicting inpatient service use among patients with bipolar affective disorder. *Psychiatric Services*, *50*, 806–812.

Physicians' Desk Reference. (2010). *Physicians' desk reference* (64th ed.). Montvale, NJ: PDR Network.

President's New Freedom Commission on Mental Health. (2003). *Achieving the promise: Transforming mental health care in America. DHHS publication number SMA-03-3832. Washington, DC: President's New Freedom Commission on Mental Health, 2003*. Retrieved from http://www.mentalhealthcommision.gov/reports/finalreport/fullreport-02.htm

Rotter, J. B. (1990). Internal versus external control of reinforcement: A case history of a variable. *American Psychologist*, *45*, 489–493. doi:10.1037/0003-066X.45.4.489

Roe, D. (2003). A prospective study on the relationship between self-esteem and functioning during the first year after being hospitalized for psychosis. *The Journal of Nervous and Mental Disease*, *191*, 45–49. doi:10.1097/00005053-200301000-00008

Seligman, M. E. P. (1995). The effectiveness of psychotherapy: The Consumer Reports Study. *American Psychologist*, *50*, 965–974. doi:10.1037/0003-066X.50.12.965

Walkup, J. T., Albano, A. M., Piacentini, J., Birmaher, B., Compton, S. N. Sherrill, J. T., . . . Kendall, P. C. (2008). Cognitive behavioral therapy, sertraline, or a combination in childhood anxiety. *The New England Journal of Medicine*, *359*, 2753–2766.

Wiggins, J. G., & Cummings, N. A. (1998). National study of the experience of psychologists with psychotropic medication and psychotherapy. *Professional Psychology: Research and Practice*, *29*, 549–552. doi:10.1037/0735-7028.29.6.549

World Health Organization. (2007). International statistical classification of diseases and related health problems: Clinical descriptions and diagnostic guidelines. Geneva, Switzerland: Author.

7

EVALUATING DRUG RESEARCH

ROBERT E. McGRATH

Pharmaceutical companies' actions in relation to research often demonstrate their vested interest in overstating the efficacy of medications.[1] Through selective presentation of results, publications of findings from drug trials often present a more positive picture of a drug's safety and efficacy than the original submission to the Food and Drug Administration (FDA; Rising, Bacchetti, & Bero, 2008). For example, a review of drug trials in which statins were compared with each other found that which company funded the study was a powerful predictor of the findings (Bero, Oostvogel, Bacchetti, & Lee, 2007). When compared with the original studies, cited findings in advertisements geared to prescribers often misrepresent findings in a manner that exaggerates the medication's usefulness (Villanueva, Peiró, Librero, & Pereiró, 2003).

Reviews of the literature and treatment guidelines, which are supposed to be based on an objective reading of the literature, are also potentially

---

[1]The efficacy of a treatment differs from its effectiveness. The former has to do with whether the medication works in tightly controlled drug trials, the latter with whether it works in the real world. This chapter focuses on studies demonstrating efficacy. Keep in mind that evidence of efficacy does not ensure effectiveness. For example, an efficacious medication with substantial side effects that reduce adherence in the real world may not be particularly effective.

tainted. One study found that 87% of practice guideline authors who responded to a survey admitted to pharmaceutical industry funding (Choudhry, Stelfox, & Detsky, 2002). In recent years the Cochrane Reviews have emerged as an important independent source of medication reviews (http://www.cochrane.org/reviews). For example, Cochrane reviews often came to more conservative conclusions about safety and efficacy than pharma-funded reviews of the same literature (Jørgensen, Hilden, & Gøtzsche, 2006). However, Cochrane reviews are still based on literature that is primarily funded by pharmaceutical companies. Even the bioethicists charged with considering the implications of such potential conflicts of interest are often funded by drug companies (Elliott, 2004).

It would be unfair to raise these concerns without acknowledging the opposing arguments. The potential for bias does not mean bias has occurred, and sometimes studies can be interpreted in different ways. When an independent source criticizes marketing practices or draws more negative conclusions about a drug than a source funded by the pharmaceutical industry, one may question whether the independent source has an antipharma bias. Even when bias has potentially occurred, it is unclear to what extent it resulted from malevolent intent versus the cognitive biases one inevitably finds in an advocate.

Though one may argue about the extent to which the available literature is biased in favor of the pharmaceutical industry, certain conclusions are unquestionable. The potential and motivation for bias exist, and the literature on cognitive bias teaches us that bias is probably inevitable. Given the systemic biological effects of pharmaceuticals, a bias in favor of the efficacy and safety of medications has potentially dangerous consequences. However, the consequences of bias can be minimized if (a) the potential for bias is recognized and (b) the person continues to test one's judgments against new data as it becomes available. To put it in more generally familiar terminology, psychologists must be critical consumers of drug research. This will require looking beyond the take-home conclusion in the abstract or advertisement and considering whether the data actually support that conclusion. This task need not take long, but it does require a continuing commitment to being a good scientist.

To help psychologists become more critical consumers of drug research, this chapter addresses several issues. The first section offers a basic review of key concepts in statistics that psychologists will need when they are reading research results. The second section applies these concepts to some real-world data and demonstrates how materials provided by drug companies can be used by the critical consumer. The final section describes some important questions to ask of any study that will help the reader look at the study more objectively.

This chapter is intended as a how-to-read-research guide rather than a how-to-do-research guide. It focuses on randomized clinical trials (RCTs), which provide much of the available data on the efficacy and safety of medications. RCTs are studies in which members of some patient population are randomly assigned to one of two or more conditions, thereby creating samples that represent two populations defined by the treatment they receive. In the two-condition case, these usually involve receiving an experimental drug or a comparison treatment. The comparison is usually a placebo but may involve no treatment or an alternate treatment such as a different drug with known efficacy.

A BASIC STATISTICAL REVIEW

Significance Testing

Significance testing remains the most popular method for drawing inferences about populations from samples. For those readers who are rusty on such matters, the logic of significance testing can be reviewed briefly as applied to an RCT of an antidepressant. You start by assuming that no difference exists in the mean improvement for the population of depressives given the experimental drug versus the population given the comparison treatment, an assumption called the null hypothesis. To use more current terminology, the null hypothesis suggests no *effect* exists in the population. You compute some sample statistic that is relevant to testing null hypotheses, such as the t statistic. The t statistic is relevant because it is possible to estimate the probability of getting a particular value for t if the null hypothesis is true. Suppose the sample t value is 2.47 and there are 15 participants in each condition ($n = 30$). It can be determined that if the null hypothesis is true, a t value at least this large should only occur in 1 out of every 100 samples, for a probability of .01. This is called the p value. You might consider this sufficiently unusual to conclude the null hypothesis is false—that is, for rejecting the null hypothesis—knowing there is still a 1 in 100 chance of getting this result if the null hypothesis is true and the drug is no better than the comparison treatment. The p value at which we are willing to make this decision to reject is called the α level. You might have decided, as most do, that an outcome as frequent as high as 5 in 100 (.05) would have justified rejecting the null hypothesis. That would mean the p value was .01 but the α level was .05, and because $p < .05$, you could reject the null hypothesis. Rejecting the null hypothesis when it is true is called a *Type I error*, so α represents the risk of a Type I error acceptable to the researcher.

Some readers of this chapter may be surprised to find that psychologists have been quite critical of significance testing as a method of drawing inferences about populations (e.g., Kline, 2004; Oakes, 1986). A good deal has been written about this issue, but two related objections to the method are relevant here. The first is that the hypothesis of no difference in the population means is almost certain to be false. Even if participants are randomly assigned under double-blind conditions, so neither the one treating nor the one treated knows whether a participant is receiving the active drug, any systematic difference in the conditions of the treatments can cause differences in the population means. In the case of psychotropic medications, for example, these drugs often have an activating effect. Users of antidepressants may notice a change in sensorium, a perception that "something is happening" internally, which creates a positive expectation. In contrast, the placebo is often completely inert. It has been suggested that as much as half of the effectiveness of antidepressants is because of this activating effect (Moncrieff, Wessely, & Hardy, 1998), which is unrelated to true antidepressant properties.

The second issue is that significance is often treated as if it indicated the importance of the finding. This is, for example, the implicit reason why many articles use one asterisk for tests where $p < .05$, two for those where $p < .01$, and so forth: There is an implication that a smaller p value suggests a more important treatment. In fact, significance testing is about whether or not the null hypothesis is true and nothing else. It is true that an effect cannot be important if it does not exist, so significance indicates something relevant to importance. However, statistical significance is perhaps a necessary but definitely not a sufficient condition for concluding that a treatment is important. For example, two drugs may both alleviate migraines better than placebo; therefore, both are efficacious. If Drug A has no serious side effects while Drug B often causes permanent liver damage, though, then finding efficacy for Drug A is more important than finding it for Drug B.

These two problems—the potential for alternative explanations for a significant finding and the tendency to equate significance with importance—are not problems with significance tests but with how people tend to use them. The use of a significant result should never be the sole basis for deciding whether the use of a medication is justified.

To evaluate whether a medication is clinically important, additional concepts are needed. Where α is the probability of rejecting the null hypothesis if the null hypothesis is true, *power*, symbolized as $1 - \beta$, is the probability of rejecting the null hypothesis if the null hypothesis is false, that is, if an effect actually exists in the population. The complement to the power of the study, β, is the probability of not rejecting the null hypothesis even though it is false: a *Type II error*. Where traditional significance testing focuses on what happens when the null hypothesis is true, considering power requires considering what happens when the null hypothesis is false.

The power of the study is a function of three factors: α (the larger the alpha, the greater the power), sample size (the larger the sample size, the greater the power), and the effect size (the larger the effect size, the greater the power). Effect size is essentially "how wrong" the null hypothesis is in a given population. If there is no effect, then the null hypothesis is correct. If the correlation between two variables in the population is .10, then the null hypothesis is wrong but not as wrong as it is if the population correlation is .30. It is easier to detect a population effect (reject the null hypothesis) if the population correlation is .30 than it is if the population correlation is .10, and it is even easier if the population correlation is .50. The correlation is one of a number of statistics that are available for estimating effect size, as will be discussed shortly.

How does this additional information contribute to deciding whether a treatment is important? Suppose we are testing a new drug for schizophrenia and find it is significantly better than a placebo. All we know so far is that the drug seems to be better than the placebo. How important this finding is, whether it justifies using this medication in practice, depends on four factors:

1. Effect size: The larger the improvement over placebo, the better the medication. The results of the significance test lead us to conclude the effect size is not zero, but they provide no further information on how large the effect size is.
2. Cost: The cheaper the active treatment, the better the medication.
3. Risks: Medications with fewer and less severe side effects are better medications.
4. Targets: The more important the symptoms targeted by the medication, the better the medication. For example, finding regular use of aspirin can reduce the frequency of heart attacks (Willard, Lange, & Hillis, 1992) represents a more important target than mild joint pain.

Notice that one factor is common to the three determinants of power and the four determinants of importance: effect size. It is for this reason that the level of significance (.05 or .01) is sometimes confused with the importance of the treatment: Larger effects are associated with both the level of significance and with the importance of the effect. More direct methods of estimating the importance of a treatment exist, though. The first step involves estimating the effect size.

Effect Size Statistics

Given the previous discussion, it is not surprising that over time psychologists have come to consider the effect size in some ways a more interesting piece of information than whether a test statistic such as *t* is significant. This recognition has been enhanced by the success of *meta-analysis*, a statistical method introduced about 40 years ago that has come to dominate literature reviews in the field. Meta-analysis usually involves averaging effect sizes across studies and using the resulting mean as a best estimate of the population effect size. Certain effect-size statistics now regularly appear in clinical research. Here are some of the more useful ones:

1. The *standardized mean difference:* This statistic is the most commonly used for gauging the size of the effect between the means of two groups. For this reason it has a particularly important role to play in drug RCTs where the dependent measure is a dimensional variable such as score or improvement on the Hamilton (1967) Depression Rating scale (HDRS). There are various formulas available for estimating the population standardized mean difference from a sample (McGrath & Meyer, 2006), but the most popular is called d:

$$d = \frac{\bar{Y}_{\cdot 1} - \bar{Y}_{\cdot 2}}{S_{pooled}}.$$

That is, the difference between the two group means is divided by the pooled standard deviation for the two groups. That means, for example, that $d = 0.50$ indicates the difference between the two means is half the size of the standard deviation.

2. The *correlation coefficient* (r): This statistic is widely familiar to psychologists as an indicator of the strength of the relationship between two dimensional variables. It can also be used to gauge the strength of the relationship between one dichotomous variable and one dimensional variable (when it is often called the *point-biserial correlation*), or between two dichotomous variables (often called the *phi coefficient*). The phi coefficient can be used, for example, in a two-condition RCT where the dependent measure is dichotomous, such as improved–unimproved or still depressed–no longer depressed. For example, the data in Table 7.1 are associated with a phi coefficient of (correlation coefficient) of .20. However, other effect-size measures have become more popular for the case of two dichotomous variables. Here are three that are particularly popular.

3. The *relative risk ratio* (RR): This statistic compares the proportion of patients improving with medication versus the proportion improving with placebo:

$$RR = \frac{n_{11}/(n_{11} + n_{12})}{n_{21}/(n_{21} + n_{22})} = \frac{14/(14 + 36)}{6/(6 + 44)} = 2.33.$$

TABLE 7.1
Symbols for 2 × 2 Tables

	Improved	Not improved
Medication	$n_{11} = 14$	$n_{12} = 36$
Placebo	$n_{21} = 6$	$n_{22} = 44$

Note. Symbols refer to the number of cases in each cell. For example, n_{11} is the number of people who improved taking the active medication. Numbers are provided to serve as the basis for demonstrating the computation of various statistics.

If there is no effect, then the proportion of patients improving is equal in both treatments and RR = 1.0. For effective treatments RR should be >1.0. For example, if the dependent measure is improved–unimproved, RR > 1.0 means the proportion improving from the active medication is larger than the proportion improving from placebo. A value of 2.33 means that a person taking the medication is 2.33 times as likely to improve as the person taking placebo. The interpretation reverses if the outcome is a negative one such as deteriorated–not deteriorated, in which case the statistic indicates the relative risk of the two procedures.

4. The *odds ratio* (OR): This statistic represents the odds of improving with medication versus the odds of improving with placebo. For the data in Table 7.1 the odds ratio is

$$OR = \frac{n_{11}/n_{12}}{n_{21}/n_{22}} = \frac{n_{11} * n_{22}}{n_{21} * n_{12}} = \frac{14 * 44}{6 * 36} = 2.85.$$

If there is no effect, then the odds for the two treatments are equal and OR = 1.0. For effective treatments OR should be >1.0. For example, if the dependent measure is improved–unimproved, OR > 1.0 means the odds of improving from the active medication is larger than the odds of improving from

TABLE 7.2
Benchmarks for Small, Medium, and Large Effect Sizes

Statistic	Effect size			
	None	Small	Medium	Large
r	0	0.10	0.30	0.50
d	0	0.20	0.50	0.80
OR	1.00	1.49	3.45	9.00
log(OR)	0	0.40	1.24	2.20
RR	1.00	1.22	1.86	3.00
NNT	∞	10.00	3.33	2.00

Note. OR = odds ratio; RR = relative risk ratio; NNT = number needed to treat.

placebo. Because a no-effect point of 1.0 is potentially confusing, researchers often report the natural log of the OR instead, so that the no-effect value is shifted to 0 as is the case for d and r.

A number of articles critical of the OR have been published (e.g., Sackett, Deeks, & Altman, 1996). Perhaps the most serious problem with this statistic is that people do not appreciate the difference between odds and the proportions used to compute relative risk. If 75 of 100 people improve on the medication, the proportion of improvement is $75/100 = 0.75$, but the odds of improving are 75 to 25 = $75/25 = 3.0$. An OR of 2.85 indicates the odds of improving are 2.85 times larger for those taking the medication than for those taking the placebo. I have seen published articles in which the authors confused the odds ratio with the risk ratio, for example, suggesting an odds ratio of 2.85 means those taking the medication are 2.85 times as likely to improve, but that is incorrect: What it means is that the odds of improvement are 2.85 times as large. I suspect this mistake occurs because people have a better intuitive grasp of relative risk than relative odds. Unfortunately, certain more complicated statistical procedures, such as logistic regression, involve the OR; therefore, it remains a popular statistic.

5. The *number needed to treat* (NNT): This statistic represents the number of cases needed to receive the active treatment to generate one more positive outcome than the comparison treatment. For example,

$$NNT = \frac{1}{n_{11}/(n_{11}+n_{12}) - n_{21}/(n_{21}+n_{22})} = \frac{1}{14/(14+36) - 6/(6+44)} = 6.25.$$

This value means that if you treat 6.25 people with the medication, you will get one more positive outcome than you would from treating those 6.25 people with placebo. NNT differs from the two previous statistics in that smaller NNT values are better. One problem with NNT is that it is scaled oddly, though the scaling makes sense in the context of the information the statistic is trying to provide. When there is no effect, so the proportion improving from medication is the same as that improving from placebo, then the denominator is 0 and NNT is infinitely large. If everyone taking medication improves and no one on placebo improves, then NNT is 1.0. Therefore, values closer to 1.0 are more desirable for positive outcomes.

The example provided in Table 7.1 demonstrates one of the important lessons to learn about commonly used effect size statistics. These statistics estimate the efficacy of medication *relative* to the alternative condition. Compared with this placebo, the medication tested in Table 7.1 was relatively more efficacious. This is a very different issue from the medication's *absolute* efficacy. Improvement occurred for substantially less than half of those who took it. This is not a criticism of the medication or the statistics: Finding that the medication is better than the placebo is a worthwhile finding. However, consumers of research often ignore the difference between absolute and relative efficacy, a lapse that can tend to encourage overestimating the likelihood of improvement in response to the medication.

Gigerenzer, Gaissmaier, Kurz-Milcke, Schwarz, and Woloshin (2008) provided a useful example of the dangers involved in focusing only on relative risk.[2] In 1995, an advisory committee in the United Kingdom issued a warning that the use of certain oral contraceptives increased the risk of potentially life-threatening blood clots by 100%, a relative risk statistic. The result was a dramatic decline in the use of such contraceptives, and it was estimated that 13,000 more abortions occurred in the following year as a result. It is questionable whether the same outcome would have resulted if it were made public that this 100% risk increase corresponded to an absolute increase in risk from 1 per 7,000 women to 2. What is particularly unfortunate in this episode is that pregnancy and abortion are both associated with a greater increase in the risk of blood clots than the use of the pill.

Cohen (1988) provided some rules of thumb for what defines a small, medium, or large effect size. These were intended only as rough heuristics, and some commentators have provided recommendations for revising these benchmarks (e.g., McGrath & Meyer, 2006), but Cohen's values remain both popular in the literature and useful as a rough gauge of effect size. Though he did not provide benchmarks for RR, OR, or NNT, these can be extrapolated from the values he provided for the correlation coefficient (see Table 7.2).

This information can directly inform judgments about the importance of a finding. For example, a treatment with high risks or minimal benefit will need to demonstrate a larger effect than a treatment with fewer risks or greater benefit for the first treatment to be an important innovation, other factors being equal. Notice that different effect size statistics need not agree on the size of an effect: Most of the statistics computed indicated the example provided in Table 7.2 is associated with a small-to-medium effect, but RR suggests a medium-to-large effect. This is a recognized problem when different effect sizes are computed (McGrath & Meyer, 2006).

Confidence Intervals

Researchers are increasingly coming to prefer *confidence intervals* (CIs) over significance testing as a strategy for drawing inferences about populations

---

[2]More generally, Gigerenzer et al. (2008) discussed the role of statistical illiteracy in health care. That topic is beyond the scope of this chapter, but their article should be required reading for all health care professionals.

from samples. Where significance testing has to do with whether the effect size is equal to zero, which I have already suggested is almost never the case, CIs have to do with estimating the size of the effect, a more interesting issue in most circumstances. A CI is a range in which some population statistic such as a mean, correlation, or odds ratio is likely to fall based on a sample. For example, a sample mean of 51.7 is the best single estimate of the population mean. It is also possible to define a 95% CI for the mean, perhaps 49.26 to 54.14. It can be demonstrated that in 95% of samples the population mean will fall within the sample's 95% CI for the mean. The CI, therefore, gives you a more reasonable guess about the population mean than the sample mean alone.

The level of confidence can vary: Common alternatives to 95% include 90 or 99, but the choice is completely up to the researcher; higher levels of confidence require wider CIs. Where the 95% interval is 49.26 to 54.14, the 90% interval is 49.65 to 53.75, whereas the 99% interval is 48.46 to 54.94. Larger samples also produce smaller CIs.

Experts in statistical analysis often recommend CIs as the best inferential strategy in the case of individual studies, and meta-analysis as the best strategy for drawing inferences across a body of literature. These recommendations increasingly influence statistical practice, and this has been particularly true in the case of drug research.

Patient Withdrawal

Another statistical issue that frequently arises in drug research involves what to do about the chronic problem of patient withdrawal. In drug trials this is often addressed by conducting one of two types of analyses. *Last observation carried forward* (LOCF) analysis means that patients are compared on their last data point no matter when it occurred. For example, suppose in a 12-week trial of an antidepressant Patient 92 withdrew after Week 4, Patient 46 withdrew after Week 8, and Patient 107 completed the trial. All three patients will be included in all analyses, using their most recent data point. For example, the comparison at Week 9 would include Patient 92's score from Week 4, Patient 46's score from Week 8, and Patient 107's score for Week 9. In contrast, observed cases (OC) analysis is restricted to those individuals who are still participating at the time of the comparison; therefore, of our three participants, only 107 would be included in the Week 9 comparison.

In studies with high dropout rates, LOCF can include substantially more individuals. One might expect that LOCF analyses are associated with smaller effect sizes than OC analyses, because the former includes participants who presumably withdrew before receiving the full benefit of the medication, but this difference in effect size does not necessarily occur (e.g., Kirsch, Moore, Scoboria, & Nicholls, 2002). Why that might be is unclear, but the result is that the LOCF analysis can be more powerful than the OC analysis. The more serious issue, because it is often impossible to determine how many cases have withdrawn when the researcher uses LOCF analyses, is that it is unclear to the reader how many data points in the 12-week comparison actually reflect 12 weeks of treatment.

APPLICATIONS

Sometimes, the most immediate problem faced by clinicians who are trying to become more critical consumers of drug research is getting access to the drug research. Although those with academic appointments often have extensive electronic access to research journals, clinicians rarely have that luxury. If you do not, the materials that pharmaceutical companies distribute at meetings or on the Internet can be extremely useful. It is presumed that the information available through these sources was chosen specifically because it is particularly supportive of the product, and as noted earlier it may be presented in such a way that it exaggerates the product's efficacy or safety (Villanueva et al., 2003). Even so, a close look at the evidence can often raise interesting questions about the claims made.

In preparation for writing this chapter I randomly selected Abilify (aripiprazole) to evaluate. An Internet search revealed the corporate website for this product (http://www.abilify.com). After a bit of browsing I found a link for "U.S. Healthcare Professionals," which led me to a link that provided evidence for the efficacy of Abilify as an adjunct to antidepressants for the treatment of bipolar I disorder and as a treatment for schizophrenia. Clicking on the first option led to a page that provided results from several studies (http://www.abilify.com/hcp/major-depressive-disorder-efficacy.aspx). A portion of the page adapted from a study reported by Berman et al. (2007) is provided in Figure 7.1.

What can we learn from Figure 7.1? First, the study focused on two groups that were given either a combination of antidepressant and Abilify ($n = 181$) or an antidepressant and a placebo ($n = 172$). Analyses were conducted on a week-by-week basis. This is an LOCF analysis, meaning all 353 participants were included in each analysis. This procedure is likely to be associated with greater power than an OC analysis, but it does not give us any information about the number who dropped out of each group at each data point.

We can see that adding aripiprazole to another antidepressant produced significant effects even at Week 2. However, given the large sample size, a medium standardized mean different in the population (.50) is associated with power of .999, whereas even a small effect (.20) is associated with power of .60. That aripiprazole was a significantly better adjunctive treatment than the placebo therefore does not tell us much about the likely size of the population

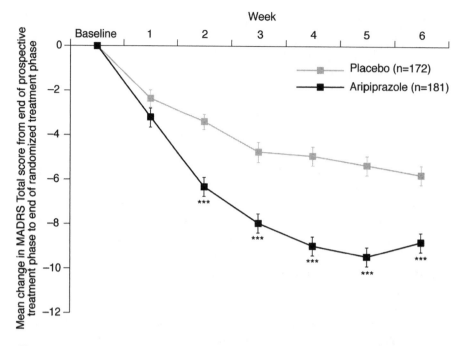

Figure 7.1. Results available at http://www.abilify.com. Adapted from "The efficacy and safety of aripiprazole as adjunctive therapy in major depressive disorder: A multicenter, randomized, double-blind, placebo-controlled study" by R. M. Berman, R. N. Marcus, R. Swanink, R. D. McQuade, W. H. Carson, P. K. Corey-Lisle, and A. Khan, A., 2007, *Journal of Clinical Psychiatry, 68,* p. 848. Copyright 2007 by Physician's Postgraduate Press, Inc. Adapted with permission.

effect, and it is the size of the effect that helps us to decide whether the effect is large enough to justify the risks and costs of a second medication.

The results provided do not allow for computation of any of the effect-size statistics summarized, though it would be possible to compute *d* if the figure included standard deviations as well as means. The closest measure possible based on what is provided is the difference between the means. At the maximum, this difference is about 4 points. Is this enough of a difference to be considered important?

To help answer that question, it is worth noting that the dependent measure here is change in score on the Montgomery–Åsberg Depression Rating scale (MADRS; Montgomery & Åsberg, 1979). A quick online search reveals it is a clinician rating scale of depression, and it is the most commonly used dependent measure in antidepressant trials with the exception of the HDRS. Copies of the instrument can be accessed online, and this is true of many of the measures commonly used in drug trials. In this way you will find the MADRS involves rating patients on 10 items. Each item is rated on a four-step scale from 0 to 6, with each step worth 2 more points than the previous step, so the MADRS total score is scaled 0 to 60.

Consider what this information reveals about the effect Abilify has when compared with the placebo as an adjunctive treatment. A 4-point difference means clinician ratings declined by only two steps across the 10 items. Is that enough of a difference to justify the additional cost and risk of a second medication? I encourage you to seek out a copy of the MADRS online and consider this question for yourself.

This exercise is not intended to suggest that the information in Figure 7.1 is misleading or inaccurate. In particular, this study is a particularly strong one in that both groups received an active antidepressant, so differences in activation between the two groups as a possible alternative explanation can be ruled out. Furthermore, it is important to keep in mind that 4 points is the mean difference. Some people may be expected to do substantially better, though some should also do substantially worse. The point is that a realistic evaluation of the enhancement that results from adding Abilify to another antidepressant reveals that the improvement can be quite minimal and far from the result that patients and practitioners may expect. It also highlights several of the principles outlined previously: A significant difference need not indicate an important difference; it is not enough to read the claims without challenging those claims; and expectations for a treatment must consider issues of cost, risks, and targets.

Not all websites are as generous about providing outcomes data as http://www.abilify.com. Another useful source for this type of information is the multicolored, glossy brochures handed out by drug company representatives at professional conferences or at prescribers' offices. Flipping past the pictures of lovers on a beach and people cherishing life, you will often find a graph or two that tells you what you need to know about the medication's efficacy. Finally, even if you do not have access to an online professional library of journals, it is often worth conducting an Internet search for the primary source article. At the worst you may decide to pay a fee for access to the article, but a surprising number will pop up for free in full-text form.

QUESTIONS TO ASK

You should ask a series of questions about any drug trial (see also Smith, 2005; Tyrer & Kendall, 2009). Asking these questions will help you be a more critical user of medications.

1. Does the article meet recommended standards for describing studies? CONsolidated Standards Of Reporting Trials (CONSORT) represents a checklist of 22 aspects of a clinical trial that should

be included in a description of the methodology (http://www.consort-statement.org). Preferred Reporting Items for Systematic Reviews and Meta-Analyses (PRISMA; http://www.prisma-statement.org), formerly called QUality Of Reporting Of Meta-analyses (QUOROM), serves the same purpose for meta-analyses, as does STAndards for the Reporting of Diagnostic (STARD; http://www.stard-statement.org) accuracy studies for studies that are attempting to classify participants into groups. These checklists are widely known, available, and accepted. If a research article fails to mention aspects of the design listed in the applicable checklist, it is worth wondering why the authors chose to do so.

2. Is there a comparison between groups?[3] If not, assume the effect is exaggerated. For practical reasons many studies use a one-group, pretest–posttest design in which all participants receive the active treatment. If the dependent measure is a variable that demonstrates substantial stability over time, this can be an efficient (and ethically superior) alternative to randomly assigning some participants to placebo. When the dependent measure is sensitive to environmental circumstances, however, this methodology tends to exaggerate the treatment effect. For example, Goldberg et al. (2007) provided evidence that improvements in cognitive functioning among first-episode schizophrenics administered second-generation antipsychotics may represent nothing more than practice effects. In a classic review of meta-analytic results that concern the effectiveness of psychosocial interventions, Lipsey and Wilson (1993) found that effect sizes from one-group, pretest–posttest designs, were 61% larger than those based on comparisons between groups.

3. If there is a significant difference between drug and placebo, are there other reasonable explanations for the finding beside the efficacy of the medication? Any factor that could result in a systematic difference between the two groups other than the targeted effect of the medication is a possible factor. Two in particular are worth considering. Open trials without blinding are inherently flawed as sources of evidence (e.g., Leucht et al., 2009). The other issue always to consider is whether the study involves an activating comparison treatment.

4. If there is a significant effect that supports the use of the medication, how large is the sample? The larger the sample size, the

---

[3] I am indebted to Robert H. Pietrzak for suggesting this topic to me.

less a significant result can be attributed to the size of the population effect. Funded drug studies typically use samples of 350 or more. They do so because FDA approval depends on demonstrating a significant difference from placebo as well as evidence of the medication's safety. With $N = 350$, even standardized mean differences of .30, which are substantially smaller than the value considered typical or medium sized, are associated with power of .80 or higher.

5. If a study reveals that some side effect occurs at the same rate whether patients are given the medication or a placebo (i.e., the study finds no significant difference), how small is the sample? The discussion in this chapter has focused on efficacy studies, but safety studies are essential to the evaluation of risk associated with the medication. Given the primary importance awarded to avoiding harm in health care decision making, a serious risk can be associated with a very small effect size and still represent essential information about a medication's risk–benefit analysis: One death due to the medication can raise serious questions about its use. If research fails to demonstrate a higher rate of a serious adverse event in the active treatment group, ask whether the sample size was large enough to detect it. To provide some context, small effects require a sample size of at least 388 before power reaches even .50, and 788 to reach .80. For very small effects ($d = 0.05$), those numbers increase from 6,000 to 12,000. What this means in practice is that a sufficiently powerful test of a medication's serious adverse effects may not occur until after the medication has received FDA approval and is marketed to millions of people. It is therefore not surprising that Lasser et al. (2002) found that warnings of serious adverse effects were added for 8% of medications after going to market, whereas 3% were withdrawn completely. If the source does not provide an effect size estimate, but you can find a t value or means and standard deviations for each group, you should be able to compute d. There are resources online that will do it for you, and it only takes a couple of minutes. Presentations of results intended primarily for marketing such as those on the Abilify website often do not provide enough information to compute d. Even so, as the discussion of Figure 7.1 demonstrated, you can still ask important questions about whether the size of the effect is large enough by treating the difference between the means as a form of effect size and considering whether that difference is big enough given the questionnaire being used.

6. What is the absolute rate of improvement? All the statistics discussed in this chapter, including t, d, OR, and the rest, evaluate change from baseline in response to the target treatment relative to that in the comparison treatment. This is important information, but it reveals only one side of the story. You should also be looking at mean change or proportion improved within those who received the active treatment, to decide whether the amount of improvement justifies the medication's use.

7. Is there a potential "file drawer problem" (Rosenthal, 1979)? This term refers to the potential for publication bias to distort the size of estimates of population effect size. In the case of drug studies, where the funding corporation can choose to publish results selectively, it is reasonable to assume that the published literature tends to exaggerate the population effect size. If your review of the literature leads you to conclude that the effect size is acceptable but not as large as would be desired, assume that the true effect size is actually somewhat smaller than the value you have computed.

8. How appropriate is the comparison condition? FDA approval requires nothing more from efficacy research than a demonstration that the drug is significantly superior to placebo, but for the clinician a more important question is how it compares with existing treatments. Even if trials compare the new medication with an existing treatment, however, it is important to consider (a) was the best alternative selected and (b) was the protocol for that alternative optimal? For example, a new medication can look safer than current treatment if the trials consistently focus on a high-potency alternative (Tyrer & Kendall, 2009) or consistently use a very high dose of the alternative. A new medication can look more efficacious than current treatment if trials focus on a low-potency alternative or implement a protocol for the alternative that is suboptimal in terms of duration or dosage. Note that Figure 7.1 provides none of the information about these very important issues; in fact, such information is rarely made available except in the original research study.

9. Is the sample appropriate? It is not necessarily the case that having rigorous criteria means the results will not generalize to other groups, but it should be a concern. In particular, by selecting individuals with a relatively low level of the disorder it is possible to generate a fairly high remission rate.

When all is said and done, many people who are suffering from psychological disorders have benefited from medications, and medication will remain an essential component of treatment. This chapter is not intended to quash the reader's enthusiasm for medication as a treatment modality. However, there are powerful entities that benefit from a health care milieu in which professionals rely too casually and consistently on medication as the treatment of choice. All prescribers have an ethical responsibility to be critical users of medications given the costs and possible risks associated with their use. Unfortunately, far too many prescribers ignore that responsibility and because of time constraints accept the information provided to them about medications at face value. Psychologists have the skills necessary to do it better; let us hope we meet that challenge.

REFERENCES

Berman, R. M., Marcus, R. M., Swanink, R., McQuade, R. D., Carson, W. H., Corey-Lisle, P. K., & Khan, A. (2007). The efficacy and safety of aripiprazole as adjunctive therapy in major depressive disorder: A multicenter, randomized, double-blind, placebo-controlled study. *The Journal of Clinical Psychiatry, 68,* 843–853. doi:10.4088/JCP.v68n0604

Bero, L., Oostvogel, F., Bacchetti, P., & Lee, K. (2007). Factors associated with findings of published trials of drug-drug comparisons: Why some statins appear more efficacious than others. *PLoS Medicine, 4,* e184. doi:10.1371/journal.pmed.0040184

Choudhry, N. K., Stelfox, H. T., & Detsky, A. S. (2002). Relationships between authors of clinical practice guidelines and the pharmaceutical industry. *JAMA, 287,* 612–617. doi:10.1001/jama.287.5.612

Cohen, J. (1988). *Statistical power analysis for the behavioral sciences* (2nd ed.). Hillsdale, NJ: Erlbaum.

Elliott, C. (2004). Six problems with pharma-funded bioethics. *Studies in History and Philosophy of Biological and Biomedical Sciences, 35,* 125–129. doi:10.1016/j.shpsc.2003.12.008

Gigerenzer, G., Gaissmaier, W., Kurz-Milcke, E., Schwartz, L. M., & Woloshin, S. (2008). Helping doctors and patients make sense of health statistics. *Psychological Science in the Public Interest, 8,* 53–96. doi:10.1111/j.1539-6053.2008.00033.x

Goldberg, T. E., Goldman, R. S., Burdick, K. E., Malhotra, A. K., Lencz, T., Patel, R. C., . . . Delbert, G. (2007). Cognitive improvement after treatment with second-generation antipsychotic medications in first-episode schizophrenia: Is it a practice effect? *Archives of General Psychiatry, 64,* 1115–1122. doi:10.1001/archpsyc.64.10.1115

Hamilton, M. (1967). Development of a rating scale for primary depressive illness. *The British Journal of Social and Clinical Psychology, 6,* 278–296.

Jørgensen, A. W., Hilden, J., & Gøtzsche, P. C. (2006, October 6). Cochrane reviews compared with industry supported meta-analyses and other meta-analyses of the same drugs: Systematic review. *British Medical Journal, 333.* doi:10.1136/bmj.38973.444699.0B.

Kirsch, I., Moore, T. J., Scoboria, A., & Nicholls, S. S. (2002, July 15). The emperor's new drugs: An analysis of antidepressant medication data submitted to the U.S. Food and Drug Administration. *Prevention & Treatment, 5,* Article 23. Retrieved from http://journals.apa.org/prevention/volume5/pre0050023a.html

Kline, R. B. (2004). *Beyond significance testing: Reforming data analysis methods in behavioral research.* Washington, DC: American Psychological Association. doi:10.1037/10693-000

Lasser, K. E., Allen, P. D., Woolhandler, S. J., Himmelstein, D. U., Wolfe, S. M., & Bor, D. H. (2002). Timing of new black box warnings and withdrawals for prescription medications. *JAMA, 287,* 2215–2220. doi:10.1001/jama.287.17.2215

Leucht, S., Corves, C., Arbter, D., Engel, R. R., Li, C., & Davis, J. M. (2009, January 3). Second-generation versus first-generation antipsychotic drugs for schizophrenia: A meta-analysis. *The Lancet, 373,* 31–41. doi:10.1016/S0140-6736(08)61764-X

Lipsey, M. W., & Wilson, D. B. (1993). The efficacy of psychological, educational, and behavioral treatment: Confirmation from meta-analysis. *American Psychologist, 48,* 1181–1209. doi:10.1037/0003-066X.48.12.1181

McGrath, R. E., & Meyer, G. J. (2006). When effect sizes disagree: The case of *r* and *d*. *Psychological Methods, 11,* 386–401. doi:10.1037/1082-989X.11.4.386

Moncrieff, J., Wessely, S., & Hardy, R. (1998). Meta-analysis of trials comparing antidepressants with active placebos. *The British Journal of Psychiatry, 172,* 227–231. doi:10.1192/bjp.172.3.227

Montgomery, S. A., & Åsberg, M. (1979). A new depression scale designed to be sensitive to change. *The British Journal of Psychiatry, 134,* 382–389. doi:10.1192/bjp.134.4.382

Oakes, M. L. (1986). *Statistical inference: A commentary for the social and behavioral sciences.* New York, NY: Wiley.

Rising, K., Bacchetti, P., & Bero, L. (2008). Reporting bias in drug trials submitted to the Food and Drug Administration: Review of publication and presentation. *PLoS Medicine, 5,* e217. doi:10.1371/journal.pmed.0050217.

Rosenthal, R. (1979). The file drawer problem and tolerance for null results. *Psychological Bulletin, 86,* 638–641. doi:10.1037/0033-2909.86.3.638

Sackett, D. L., Deeks, J. J., & Altman, D. G. (1996). Down with odds ratios! *Evidence-Based Medicine, 1,* 164–166.

Smith, R. (2005). Medical journals are an extension of the marketing arm of pharmaceutical companies. *PLoS Medicine, 2,* e138. doi:10.1371/journal.pmed.0020138.

Tyrer, P., & Kendall, T. (2009, January 3). The spurious advance of antipsychotic drug therapy. *The Lancet, 373,* 4–5. doi:10.1016/S0140-6736(08)61765-1

Villanueva, P., Peiró, S., Librero, J., & Pereiró, I. (2003, January 4). Accuracy of pharmaceutical advertisements in medical journals. *The Lancet, 361,* 27–32. doi:10.1016/S0140-6736(03)12118-6

Willard, J. E., Lange, R. A., & Hillis, L. D. (1992). The use of aspirin in ischemic heart disease. *The New England Journal of Medicine, 327,* 175–181.

III

SETTINGS AND POPULATIONS

8

IN THE PRIVATE PRACTICE SETTING: A SURVEY OF THE EXPERIENCES OF PRESCRIBING PSYCHOLOGISTS

ELAINE S. LEVINE AND JACK WIGGINS

The evolution of private practice in psychology can be seen as a series of five major steps forward. The first was the Taft–Hartley Act, enacted in 1947 to meet the unplanned-for and dramatic increase in demand for health care created by returning veterans of World War II. Taft–Hartley was based on prepaid private health insurance plans that were funded by the employers as a tax-deductible benefit to workers and managed by the workers' union. Regrettably, standard health insurance contracts specifically excluded coverage for nervous and mental disorders, alcoholism, and tuberculosis as incurable conditions. Barriers to insuring these health conditions were eventually overcome when insurance plans for federal employees began to offer coverage for mental conditions on a trial basis in the late 1950s.

The second major step toward private practice in psychology was the 50+ years of battle it took to achieve licensure for psychologists in all 50 states, beginning with Dr. Karl Heiser's efforts that culminated in the passage of the first Psychology Certification Act in Connecticut of 1947.

The third step occurred with the inclusion of psychologists in health insurance contracts. Thanks to Drs. A. E. "Gene" Shapiro and "Maury" Goodman in 1967 (Shapiro, Dorken, Rodgers, & Wiggins, 1976), New Jersey became the first state to define psychologists as "physicians" for reimbursement in health insurance contracts and to require health insurers to offer their beneficiaries a choice of psychologists or psychiatrists for the treatment of mental disorders.

The fourth step involved obtaining hospital privileges for psychologists. The Joint Commission for the Accreditation of Hospitals (JCAH; now the Joint Commission on Accreditation of Healthcare Organizations) considered psychology to be an ancillary profession and ineligible for hospital staff membership. In 1979, Dr. Jack Wiggins, joined by the Ohio Psychological Association, filed an antitrust suit against JCAH through the Ohio Attorney General. JCAH settled the complaint in 1982 by agreeing to comply with state laws that govern hospital staff. Dr. Herbert Dorken lobbied for a hospital practice bill in California, making it the first state with hospital privileges for psychologists.

The fifth and most recent step in the process has been the acquisition of prescriptive authority. Drs. Elaine LeVine and Mario Marquez spearheaded efforts to pass the first state law authorizing psychologists to prescribe psychotropic medications for their patients in 2002 in New Mexico, a milestone soon matched in Louisiana. Though these currently remain the only two states in which psychologists can prescribe as private practitioners, they set an enormous precedent for the future of psychological private practice. Accordingly, this chapter presents results from the first survey ever conducted on the impact of prescriptive authority on private practice.

METHOD

The first step in conducting research in regard to the exigencies of prescribing in private practice involved learning more about the nature of the current independent practices of those prescribing in New Mexico and Louisiana. An open-ended oral interview format was used so that the range of independent practice approaches could be fully explored. Interview questions were designed to explore the psychologists' views on the relevance and appropriateness of their training, changes in relationships with colleagues, practical and financial aspects of practice related to prescribing, and the perceived advantages and disadvantages of being able to prescribe.

Lists of prescribing and medical psychologists were gleaned from the New Mexico Board of Psychologist Examiners and the Louisiana Board of Psychologist Examiners. Through discussion with colleagues who were instrumental in the prescriptive authority movement in each of these states, who knew the varied persons prescribing in their state, the prescribing–medical psychologists in private practice were identified. Of the 18 prescribing psychologists in New Mexico at the time of the inquiry in fall 2008, nine were identified as maintaining a part- or full-time private practice. Of the 41 medical psychologists in Louisiana at that time, 14 were identified as maintaining a part- or full-time private practice. Each of the prescribing–medical psychologists identified to be in private practice were emailed a request for their participation in a telephone interview and asked to schedule an interview.

RESULTS AND DISCUSSION

All nine of the prescribing psychologists in New Mexico in full- or part-time private practice agreed to participate in the interview. Of the 14 medical psychologists in Louisiana identified in private practice, eight participated, for a total sample of 17. The psychologists' verbatim responses in the interview were recorded. The responses were later organized into thematic categories.

Table 8.1 lists the questions asked of each interviewee. Underneath each of these questions, the common themes in responses are listed with an indication of the number and percentage of respondents from each state whose response echoed that theme.

Table 8.1 reveals some striking common viewpoints among the prescribers in New Mexico and Louisiana but also a range of differences. Some of the differences are because of the variety of practice settings (e.g., full- or part-time, rural or city, needs of the community), whereas other differences seem to reflect philosophical preferences. Regardless of these differences, there is general agreement across prescribers that their training met their expectations and also enabled them to successfully meet the needs of the patients they serve.

In general, respondents agreed that their capacity to prescribe allows them to provide higher quality, more integrated care. They listed many other benefits to prescribing as well. A number of respondents mentioned the benefits of prescribing to patients: that the care is more immediate, less expensive, and that they can reach more seriously ill patients. The psychologists stressed that an important asset of being a prescribing–medical psychologist is the authority to reduce and remove medications of limited efficacy or of a high side effect profile and, instead, to select a single, more efficacious medication that replaces polypharmacy. The right to unprescribe has greatly improved their patients functioning. One psychologist noted that he used the right to prescribe as a tool to keep patients coming in until their psychotherapy was truly completed. In other words, he believed that having the power to prescribe allowed him to also provide more thorough psychotherapy. Several others noted the advantage to themselves that resulted from a perceived enhancement in the public image of the profession. In addition, to their responses to specific interview questions, the psychologists shared fascinating anecdotes about

TABLE 8.1
Summary of Interview Themes From Medical–Prescribing Psychologists in Private Practice

Questions and response themes	LA		NM	
	n	%	n	%
What prompted you to decide to take RxP training?				
To increase expertise in area of interest, felt I could not be competent without knowing this material.	4	50	8	89
Expand services to the underserved population.	1	13	2	22
Ready for a new challenge, "They said I could not do it."	0	0	3	33
Important for the future or psychology.	2	25	0	0
Wanted to provide full service.	1	13	1	11
Interferes with competent practice if you cannot prescribe.	1	13	1	11
Wanted more respect to distinguish myself from master's level practitioners.	0	0	1	11
What did you expect from RxP training?				
To prepare me to prescribe.	4	50	5	56
To gain knowledge to apply to all patients.	2	25	4	44
Has RxP training prepared you for independent practice as a prescribing–medical psychologist?				
Yes	4	50	3	33
No	0	0	0	0
Yes, if you include the practicum.	0	0	3	33
Partly, would like more medical training.	1	13	1	11
Yes, but a lot of excess information.	1	13	1	11
Yes, but I also went to an offshore medical school.	0	0	1	11
Pretty much, but could be "torqued up" some.	1	13	0	0
Yes, but it was an eye opener to learn how much of prescribing was hype.	0	0	1	11
What is the nature of your private practice?				
Solo	5	63	9	100
Partnership	3	38	0	0
How long have you been prescribing?				
No longer prescribing.	1	13	0	0
1 year	0	0	3	33
2 years	1	13	2	22
3 years	6	75	4	44
How many patients do you treat per week?				
0–10	1	13	1	11
11–20	1	13	0	0
21–30	1	13	3	33
≥31	5	63	4	44
For what percentage of your private practice population are you prescribing?				
0–30	0	0	0	0
31–40	1	13	0	0
41–50	1	13	1	11
51–60	1	13	2	22
61–70	1	13	0	0
71–80	2	25	2	22
81–90	0	0	1	11
≥91	1	13	3	33

TABLE 8.1
Summary of Interview Themes From Medical–Prescribing
Psychologists in Private Practice   *(Continued)*

Questions and response themes	LA		NM	
	n	%	*n*	%
Of these, what percentage are you seeing for psychotherapy and medication management combined?				
0–10	0	0	1	11
11–30	0	0	0	0
31–40	0	0	1	11
41–50	0	0	0	0
51–60	0	0	2	22
61–90	0	0	0	0
≥91	5	63	4	44
What percentage are you seeing for medication management alone?				
0–10	5	63	4	44
11–20	0	0	0	0
21–30	0	0	1	11
31–50	0	0	0	0
51–60	0	0	2	22
61–70	0	0	1	11
71–90	0	0	0	0
≥91	1	13	0	0
Has the nature of your patient population changed since you have been prescribing? If so, in what ways has it changed?				
More disturbed psychologically and more comorbid psychological and medical conditions.	5	63	8	89
Practice is growing.	0	0	2	22
More personality disorders.	1	13	0	0
Psychologist is more selective in clients accepted.	1	13	0	0
More patients who were previously misdiagnosed.	0	0	2	22
More Medicaid patients.	0	0	2	22
More referrals from primary care physicians (PCPs)	1	13	2	22
More referrals from mental health professionals.	1	13	0	0
Able to do more thorough therapy and extended care because patients are stabilized on medication.	1	13	0	0
Treating more referrals from nearby military base.	1	13	0	0
Treating a prison population.	0	0	1	11
No change.	0	0	1	11
Have any PCPs refused to allow you to prescribe the medication you felt was most appropriate?				
No, they really appreciate the calls.	2	25	8	89
Yes, about 10% of the time.	3	38	0	0
Yes, a couple times.	1	13	1	11
At nursing homes the physician in charge must write the script.	0	0	1	11
Yes, a problem consulting in hospitals as the attending physician is often not the PCP and is wary of cosigning prescriptions.	1	13	0	0

(continues)

TABLE 8.1
Summary of Interview Themes From Medical–Prescribing
Psychologists in Private Practice   *(Continued)*

Questions and response themes	LA		NM	
	n	%	*n*	%
If so, how did you handle this situation?				
Give name of another potential PCP and patient followed up.	3	38	0	0
Referred to psychiatrist.	2	25	0	0
PCP continued to prescribe and psychologist provided psychotherapy only.	2	25	0	0
Not prescribing, patient did not return.	0	0	1	11
What do you see as the benefits of this collaborative relationship?				
Better integration of care for patients.	3	38	6	67
PCPs are often surprised but appreciative of the contact; good public relations.	1	13	4	44
Better monitoring of patients' physical states.	1	13	1	11
Get more referrals from PCPs	0	0	2	22
An opportunity to educate PCPs about patients.	0	0	1	11
Facilitates PCPs seeing psychologists as medical providers.	1	13	0	0
Increases patient trust and comfort about care.	1	13	0	0
Do you see any drawbacks to it?				
Logistic constraints, time consuming, delay in treatment.	7	88	4	44
Lack of standardization in implementing the collaborative agreement.	2	25	1	11
Many PCPs not really interested in collaborating, are not looking at records, giving pro forma agreement.	1	13	1	11
For someone with absolutely no medical conditions, the psychologist should not have to call in advance.	1	13	1	11
Difficulty in hospitals and nursing homes as the physician must sign.	1	13	1	11
Would do it anyway when appropriate and mandated consensus is unnecessarily burdensome.	1	13	0	0
Are you able to charge more per session? Please describe.				
Small increase.	3	38	5	56
Considerably more money because only providing fee for service.	3	38	3	33
Considerably more money because of raising rates.	4	50	1	11
Considerably more money because obtained contracts at rate similar to psychiatrists.	1	13	3	33
Have lost money in some cases, as seeing more Medicaid clients.	0	0	2	22
Less no-shows because patients need medication.	1	13	0	0
Considerably more because seeing more patients per hour for medication management.	1	13	0	0
What new costs have you incurred?				
State and federal prescribing licenses.	4	50	3	33
Liability insurance raised by about 15%.	4	50	3	33
More continuing education training is more costly because so specialized.	0	0	4	44
Significantly more unbillable time (e.g., phone calls, record keeping).	2	25	2	22

TABLE 8.1
Summary of Interview Themes From Medical–Prescribing
Psychologists in Private Practice   *(Continued)*

Questions and response themes	LA		NM	
	n	%	*n*	%
Online prescribing program and upgraded note-taking material.	2	25	1	11
Increased staffing costs (may hire a nurse).	2	25	0	0
More books.	0	0	2	22
More mileage costs for consulting at rural sites.	0	0	1	11
Cabinet for samples.	1	13	0	0
More diagnostic tests.	0	0	1	11
Has supervision by managed care changed? If so, in which ways?				
Several companies in New Mexico will not pay when a psychologist holds a conditional license.	0	0	9	100
Not generally.	3	38	6	67
A lot of trouble getting managed care to pay for the prescribing.	1	13	1	11
One insurance company wrote that they would consider it fraud if the psychologist prescribed for the patients while he held a conditional license.	0	0	1	11
One insurance carrier tries to force chronic patients into short medication management sessions.	0	0	1	11
Are you using health and behavioral codes? Are you getting reimbursed through them?				
No	7	88	8	89
Yes	0	0	1	11
Occasionally	1	13	0	0
What is your relationship with the pharmaceutical companies? Are you being visited by pharmaceutical representatives? If so, how much time do you spend with them? Do they leave you samples? Are they giving you gifts? Please describe.				
Do not come at all.	0	0	5	56
Come infrequently.	5	63	3	33
Leave samples.	4	50	0	0
Leave gifts.	4	50	0	0
Get samples from supervisor of conditional license.	0	0	1	11
Ascribe to www.nofreelunch.org	0	0	1	11
Psychiatrists in office get samples.	1	13	0	0
How do you cover telephone calls from patients on a 24-hour basis?				
Take my own calls through answering service.	6	75	4	44
Take calls on my cell phone; some have a special cell phone.	2	25	4	44
Share with supervising physician for the conditional license.	0	0	2	22
Share with another prescribing psychologist.	1	13	1	11
Have a nurse practitioner collaborating who shares call.	0	0	1	11
At nursing home consulting, share with physicians.	0	0	1	11

(continues)

Questions and response themes	LA		NM	
	n	%	*n*	%
What provisions do you make to assure the accuracy of your prescriptions?				
Write the prescription on pad with duplicate copy as well as keep written note in records.	3	38	6	67
Write prescription in chart and on a central list in office by date and person that is checked against files.	2	25	1	11
Online prescribing increases accuracy.	3	38	0	0
Dictate in front of patient; also write a note and give patient the script.	2	25	0	0
Have patient read it back to me.	0	0	1	11
Write note immediately and in clinical note detailed after session.	0	0	1	11
Write prescription on pad and keep the computerized record.	0	0	1	11
Are you doing online prescribing?				
Yes	3	38	1	11
No	3	38	8	89
How often do you run computerized drug interaction studies?				
For every client.	1	13	5	56
Frequently, especially when patient is on multiple medications.	4	50	2	22
Only occasionally, as I think I know most of the interactions.	1	13	1	11
Tend to use texts instead.	0	0	1	11
Has RxP changed your record keeping practices?				
Take more extensive notes.	5	63	3	33
For each prescription, therapist and patient sign and date that prescription has been discussed including benefits and risks.	0	0	4	44
More on computer, including scan and lab reports.	3	38	2	22
Extensive more informed consent.	2	25	2	22
Patient completes symptom rating scales.	0	0	2	22
How do you describe your relationship with pharmacists? Are they responsive, respectful?				
Excellent, they help monitor mistakes, and they are a great source of information.	8	100	9	100
What do you see as the greatest difficulties and hindrances of becoming a prescribing–medical psychologist?				
Broadened oversight of patient care, including medication effects, is a weighty responsibility.	6	75	4	44
The collaborative clause is time consuming.	4	50	2	22
Insurance problems.	0	0	3	33
Expectations of patients about medications are too high.	0	0	2	22
Increased liability risks.	1	13	1	11
Record keeping, review of lab reports is very time consuming.	2	25	1	11
Monitoring that one does not overprescribe, "need to remember we are psychologists first."	1	13	1	11

TABLE 8.1
Summary of Interview Themes From Medical–Prescribing
Psychologists in Private Practice *(Continued)*

Questions and response themes	LA		NM	
	n	%	*n*	%
Increased need for staff.	1	13	0	0
Cannot treat all those requesting help.	1	13	0	0
What do you see as the greatest advantages of becoming a prescribing–medical psychologist?				
Provide better quality, more integrated care.	7	88	5	56
Less expensive, more integrated timely care for patients.	3	38	3	33
Help stop overprescribing and rampant polypharmacy.	1	13	4	44
Enhance psychologists' professional image, empowerment with other professionals.	1	13	2	22
Better patient trust and compliance.	1	13	1	11
Through consultant work, more opportunity for overall oversight of patient care.	1	13	1	11
Can do deeper work with patients.	1	13	0	0
Freedom from managed care.	1	13	0	0
Impact a lot more seriously ill patients.	1	13	0	0

Note. LA = Louisiana; NM = New Mexico; RxP = prescriptive authority of psychologists.

their interactions with their patients. The specific responses to the interview questions and anecdotes are summarized next.

Most of the psychologists who were interviewed emphasized that the right to prescribe increases their sense of responsibility, because prescribing medication creates additional concern about patients' safety and welfare. For example, the first author, Elaine LeVine, described an experience that could be viewed as countertransference related to the responsibility of prescribing. Shortly after gaining her license to prescribe, she began treating a 40-year-old man with many medical problems who presented with a severe anxiety disorder. Among his medical problems were multiple pulmonary emboli in the lungs and leg that were treated with a blood thinner. Naturally, the patient was very anxious about his medical condition. In addition, he understood that many medications interacted with the blood thinner. Several trials with antidepressants had failed because the patient was so hypervigilant to any subtle bodily reactions that he would quickly terminate the medication. For example, he once took a 10 mg tablet of Paxil and called the psychologist within minutes to say that he could not breathe. The reactions appeared to be anxiety related because when it was explained to him that in that short time frame the medication could not have been fully metabolized, he began to relax and started breathing normally again.

The patient was then prescribed a very low dose of clonazepam to reduce his general anxiety. He called the psychologist in the middle of the night the very first evening he took this medication. He said that he was desperate because he was unable to sleep and wanted to know if he could take 5 mg of zolpidem given to him by his primary care physician (PCP) with .5 mg of clonazepam just prescribed. The psychologist needed to weigh the potential interactions, especially given that the blood thinner increases the active concentration of both zolpidem and clonazepam. After checking several references, the patient was informed he could take both medications and was asked to call the psychologist in the morning. In the morning, the patient reported that he was feeling "excellent" after a "great night's sleep." However, the psychologist was fitful all night worrying about her decision. She realized that she had reacted to his generalized anxiety. The responsibility of prescribing the medication had compounded her countertransference reaction. In that regard, the medication itself could be considered a transference object, and prescribing medication increases the gravity of the patient's and psychologist's shared responsibilities.

Despite the weight of this increased responsibility, the psychologists who responded to the survey emphasized the benefit of being able to better empower their patients and feeling more empowered as helpers. In particular, several psychologists noted cases in which their psychological skills in assessment allowed them to make better diagnoses than previous persons in charge of their patients' medication management. Because of their more accurate diagnoses, they were better able to select the appropriate medication. For example, one psychologist cited the case of a 68-year-old woman who had been treated with escitalopram for an agitated depression characterized by extreme insomnia and recurring thoughts. When her symptoms became worse, her PCP doubled the dosage of escitalopram. In contrast, the psychologist recognized this patient's need for a more calming, sedating medication. Through the clinical history, the psychologist assessed that the increase in Lexapro had actually exacerbated her sleeping disorder. When the antidepressant was switched to 30 mg of Remeron, the patient improved immediately. Similarly, a number of the psychologists shared cases in which they reported patient's success by clarifying a diagnosis and modifying medication accordingly.

It is interesting to note that most of the prescribing–medical psychologists indicated that the nature of the population they serve has changed since they began prescribing. They reported treating a more complicated population, with multiple diagnoses including medical illness, substance abuse, and physical illness. Related to this factor, the prescribing–medical psychologists noted increased referrals from PCPs and directly from psychiatric hospitals, and increased opportunities for contracts servicing underserved populations in prisons, the military, nursing homes, and rural health clinics. This finding confirms the professional expectation that prescribing psychologists in private practice will address the public needs for specialty mental health care. It also confirms the assertion that prescribing will expand the practice of psychology.

However, the prescribing did not change the way that psychologists practice because prescribing psychologists reported they saw very few patients solely for medication management, as discussed later in this chapter.

The finding that the prescribing–medical psychologists in independent practice are expanding the populations that they serve could have significant implications for future training. These findings also suggest the possible need for further specialty training for the prescribing–medical psychologist in independent practice. Many of them are now seeing patients with severe mental illness who are no longer hospitalized and at least partially functional through the careful titration of their medications. Of course, this ability to live in the community enhances the quality of their lives and reduces cost. In the past, treatment of the seriously ill was the domain of psychiatry. The prescribing–medical psychologists require expertise in all aspects of treating the severely mentally ill.

The prescribing–medical psychologists mentioned several difficulties associated with prescribing: more time needed for nonbillable record keeping, consulting with PCPs, and returning patient calls; increased costs for licenses, insurance, advanced continuing-education (CE) training, billing, and online prescribing programs; and frustrations with insurance companies in regard to their lack of familiarity with psychologists as prescribers. Specifically, a common frustration with insurance companies involved not being remunerated appropriately for medication management. Some managed care insurers are not recognizing prescribing–medical psychologists. For example, a large managed care insurer in New Mexico will not reimburse psychologists during the 2 years they hold a conditional license. Among those managed care and insurance companies that are reimbursing prescribing–medical psychologists, most do not reimburse at the same rate as psychiatrists but instead pay a rate closer to that of nurses or physician assistants.

Another area of frustration with insurance companies is that the prescribing–medical psychologists must now work with formulary limitations, which are designed to keep down the cost of medication but can interfere with providing the most efficacious medication to a patient. One psychologist described the experience as "surrealistic" whenever he dealt with a particular managed care company to obtain prior authorization to prescribe medication not on their formulary. This psychologist once spent 45 min on the phone trying to get to the right person who could authorize a medication. When finally speaking to the correct administrator, the psychologist was prepared to offer an extended explanation of why the particular medication was preferred. However, the administrator only wanted to know the identifying data of the insured. Therefore, the entire authorization process was perfunctory and appeared to be set up for the explicit purpose of discouraging and bottle-necking the use of off-formulary medications rather than checking on the appropriateness of those medications. One psychologist in New Mexico explained that a large state-managed care company was trying to force her into practicing within the traditional medical model. She was disallowed payment for psychotherapy with medication management for several patients with chronic depression and bipolar disorder and instead was restricted to 15 min or 30 min for medication management checks.

Several open-ended questions presented to the interviewees elicited very mixed responses. The prescribing–medical psychologists saw many benefits but also many problems, associated with the mandatory collaboration with the patient's PCP written into the New Mexico and Louisiana prescribing acts. In New Mexico, psychologists must collaborate with the PCP before prescribing medication unless the patient's need for a psychotropic is critical (in which case, there is a 48-hr period in which to contact the PCP after prescribing) or in a disaster area (in which case, the on-call physician can serve in the role of the PCP). The New Mexico law and regulations do not specify that the collaborating physician must agree with the psychologist's recommendation, and regulations allow for the psychologist to present an overall plan to the collaborating physician rather than to contact the physician about each change in medication. In contrast, the Louisiana law and regulations call for consultation, collaboration, and *concurrence* before the psychologist can prescribe. The interviewees reported many benefits to this collaborative relationship, including better integration of care, appreciation by the PCP of the contact, more referrals from the PCP, better monitoring of the patient's physical states, and an opportunity to educate the PCP about the patient and the services offered by psychologists. However, the prescribing–medical psychologists broadly agreed that the collaborative relationship is very time consuming and, at times, quite impractical. In fact, one psychologist in Louisiana, who stated that he very much appreciated his training and continued to believe that prescriptive authority for psychologists was a good idea, reported that the collaborative relationship, especially the concurrence clause, and economic exigencies had been so complicated for him that he was not presently prescribing. A number mentioned that, not infrequently, the PCP does not seem that interested in the collaboration. For example, physicians may listen without even having patient records in front of them. Other respondents pointed out that it seems unnecessary to call a PCP if a patient has absolutely no medical conditions.

Psychologists in several settings in Louisiana explained that the concurrence requirement has been a hindrance to providing good care. In one community, physicians had been warned that collaborating with a medical psychologist will increase their liability, with the result that some PCPs have refused to discuss a patient's medication with a psychologist. Several other psychologists indicated difficulties obtaining collaboration, concurrence, or both within hospital and nursing home settings. In some of these settings in Louisiana, the on-call physician must cosign prescriptions for psychotropics, and they are sometimes hesitant to do so. In summary, while the responding prescribing–medical psychologists believed that the collaboration with the PCP ensures better integration of care and builds trust and alliance among patients, psychologists, and physicians, many psychologists reported that because of practical constraints, it would be better to allow the prescribing–medical psychologist to consult as he or she deems appropriate.

The prescribing–medical psychologists also expressed a variety of opinions about their relationship with pharmaceutical companies. By far, the majority of the prescribing–medical psychologists are visited infrequently or not at all by pharmaceutical representatives. The primary explanation offered for psychologists not being "detailed" is the absence of a system for identifying this new set of prescribers through the pharmaceutical provider banks. Other possibilities offered were lack of access to psychologists who were practicing in rural areas or relatively small numbers of patients seen per week.

Nevertheless, the prescribers generally agreed that their ability to practice is enhanced if they have samples. Some have been able to obtain samples through partnerships and consultative relationships with psychiatrists and hospitals or through their supervising physicians. Interviewees pointed out the fine tuning that is necessary to determine appropriate psychotropic intervention is facilitated with samples so that medications can be increased or switched without significant inconvenience and cost to patients. Some emphasized that the samples increase their ability to provide care to economically distressed patients. The prescribers pointed out that subtle chemical differences in related medications can lead to very different responses in patients. When patients must purchase medications, the prescribing–medical psychologists are constrained in trying a range of options to obtain maximum effectiveness. In addition, another psychologist explained that he is committed to starting with very low dosages of medications and titrating up very gradually. It is much easier to do this with samples than to try to write a prescription that allows for this very gradual titration.

One comment by authorities who argue against prescribers using samples is that drug detailers only offer samples of the newest, most expensive medications (see Symm, Averitt, Forjuoh, & Preece, 2006). When the prescriber relies on these samples, patients may then be slotted into more expensive care. Several of the prescribing–medical psychologists countered this argument by stating that once a particular medication was established through samples as the most efficacious one, they could then attempt to switch to a related generic medication if necessary.

The prescribing–medical psychologists are acutely aware of the ongoing research about how prescribers are influenced by the gifts of pharmaceutical representatives. In fact, one psychologist indicated that he had joined an association attempting to educate patients and providers about this undesirable influence on prescribing practices. However, most of the prescribing–medical psychologists are adamant that it would not be appropriate at this time for the American Psychological Association (APA) to set up restrictive guidelines about their relationship with pharmaceutical representatives because they believe that the prescribing–medical psychologists need more time and experience to find the right balance of collaboration and skepticism in their relationships with pharmaceutical representatives.

The psychologists noted moderate cost increases. Their liability insurance has risen 15%. They must now pay for State Controlled Substance Registration ($60 annually in New Mexico and $20 annually in Louisiana) and for Federal Drug Enforcement Administration licenses (at an initial cost of $551 plus $551 to renew it every 3 years). The CE training can be more expensive because pursuing specialized content can require more travel. Several have purchased online prescribing programs with initial costs up to $1,000 and additional upgrade costs.

About half of the interviewees stated that their income had increased significantly. The increase was due, in part, to the psychologists' gaining new contracts to provide service part-time in prisons and state health and mental health facilities. In highly underserved areas, the prescribing–medical psychologists on contract indicated that they are receiving a salary commensurate with psychiatrists. A number of psychologists reported that their referral base has increased significantly since prescribing so that they can exclusively charge a fee for service, at a higher fee. Those in private practice who serve a patient population drawn from the managed care pool reported only a slight increase in fees of about $10 to $15 per session. Even so, these slight increases on an annualized basis can represent from $15,000 to $22,500 in additional income. Such an increase can more than offset any increased practice cost in prescribing, such as those mentioned previously.

Given that the prescribing–medical psychologists have indicated that they are seeing a more seriously disturbed population with medical complications, one might have expected them to be using more of the health and behavioral codes that have been made available to psychologists. At the time of the writing of this chapter, many of the psychologists interviewed were not yet aware of how to use these codes. In several cases, psychologists reported they had tried to use these codes but some managed care companies refused to pay for them or reimbursed at a very low rate. The disparities in reimbursement for these codes is an unmet advocacy and training need among psychologists, though it is one that is not confined to prescribing psychologists.

The interview data also shed light on the way psychologists are practicing psychopharmacology. By far, the majority of the prescribing–medical psychologists who were interviewed are in solo practices, but a few are in partnerships with other prescribing psychologists, other medical providers, or both.

Most of the psychologists assumed sole responsibility for all their off-hour telephone calls. Several of those in partnerships reported that they share the responsibility for after-hour calls with their partners. For a number of the psychologists, these calls are filtered through an answering service. Others take the calls directly on their cell phones. One indicated he has a special cell phone number for just this purpose. It is interesting to note that the psychologists agreed that their prescribing has not significantly increased the number of after-hour telephone calls. Several of the psychologists believed that the after-hour phone calls were minimized by their tendency to titrate medication up slowly and keep a careful watch on effects and side effects through frequent sessions. Several psychologists request that their patients call them a day or two after starting a new medication. In that way, they are able to monitor any potential problems in a proactive fashion. The psychologists thought that the time spent in very extensive, informed consent also minimized after-hour phone calls. In general, the psychologists have adopted a style in which they approach their patients as intelligent and informed consumers. Many give patients written information about the drug effects and side effects. Others have them sign an agreement in which they state they understand the effects and potential side effects of the medication.

The prescribing–medical psychologists emphasized biopsychosocial interventions, combining psychotherapy with the medication management. Most of the psychologists indicated that they rarely provide medication management without adjunctive psychotherapy, and they usually do so only for colleagues in their offices or with whom they work very closely. Several commented that they did not find medication management alone satisfactory. Because it involves less relationship with the patient, compliance is more difficult to achieve. For example, the psychologist who asks patients to telephone her about the effects of new medication indicated that patients she sees for psychotherapy are quite compliant with this request but patients she has seen for medication management alone are less compliant. Another psychologist commented that if the referral comes from psychologists who were not fully trained in psychopharmacology, the referring clinicians may not monitor the behaviors and symptoms adequately. Only one of the prescribing–medical psychologists who were interviewed is treating patients primarily for medication management and referring patients to other providers for psychotherapy. This psychologist indicated that the tremendous demand for medication management in his community has prompted his decision to practice in this way.

A number of those interviewed, including the present first author, were particularly interested in how the psychologist's prescribing influences the therapeutic relationship. One interviewee practices part time in New Mexico as a prescribing psychologist and part time in another state where he cannot prescribe. He felt significantly hampered and believed he is not able to provide nearly as good a service when he cannot prescribe. The prescribing–medical psychologists reported that they believe their prescribing is integrated into the therapy in a way that is generally different than those ascribing to the traditional medical model. They spoke about more detailed informed consent, including giving the patient more information about drugs and more collaboration with the patient about choices of drugs. Setting boundaries takes on new dimensions when interacting with patients with addictive problems. The present first author (LeVine & Orabano Mantell, 2007) wrote about how patients' psychological issues are projected on the medication and that compliance can be increased when this is carefully analyzed.

The psychologists also reported that their record keeping has changed. As mentioned previously, the respondents emphasized the increased sense of responsibility for client welfare they experience now that they are prescribing. Although using different modes, these psychologists are taking many steps to ensure the accuracy of their prescriptions. Some write their prescriptions on duplicate pads, as well as writing the prescription recommendation in their case notes. Others keep a central list of prescriptions with the office staff who check that list against written prescriptions. One psychologist asks the patient to read the prescription back to him. A number are beginning to use online prescribing programs that send the prescription directly to the pharmacy. Checks and balances are incorporated into such programs to help ensure accuracy. Another psychologist lists all the patient's medications on the front page of his paper files to be updated at each session. The respondents reported more extensive record keeping in other ways, including writing lengthier notes, integrating lab reports into clinical material, giving patients written information about drugs and having them sign an informed consent form, and having patients complete symptom checklists at each session so that they can more carefully monitor the efficacy of the medications.

The psychologists make extensive use of materials for monitoring drug interactions. The majority of the prescribing–medical psychologists check for drug interactions via computer every time there is a medication change. A minority reported that they refer to written texts to monitor the drug interactions. Another small minority stated that they felt they knew most of the drug interactions well enough for their limited formulary that they only occasionally need to check sources.

The prescribing–medical psychologists were also asked several questions about whether their training prepared them for their practice. The majority mentioned that they were drawn to study prescriptive authority because of a long-term interest in the mind–body connection. A number stated that when they began training, they did not intend to prescribe but rather were seeking new intellectual challenges and knowledge to better assist all of their patients. The psychologists interviewed had obtained their training through a variety of institutions, including Alliant University, Fairleigh Dickinson University, the Chicago School of Professional Psychology, and The Southwestern Institute for the Advancement of Psychotherapy/New Mexico State University. All believed that their training prepared them adequately to prescribe, although several said they would have liked more direct training in medicine, and one thought that he received much more training than was necessary to be a safe prescriber. The psychologists in New Mexico emphasized how much they felt they had gained from their practicum experiences, which are not required for licensure in Louisiana.

CONCLUSION

With the passage of prescriptive authority laws in New Mexico and Louisiana, psychology has forged an opening in the last remaining scope of practice barrier that impedes psychology from becoming a full-service mental health care profession. Findings from the present descriptive study, based on interview data of prescribing–medical psychologists in New Mexico and Louisiana, offer hope that the authority to prescribe, as well as to not prescribe or unprescribe, is providing an avenue whereby psychologists are viewed as full-fledged primary care providers. Further, we now have some data to respond to the debate about whether or not psychologists should prescribe and whether they can do so safely and effectively.

The results from this preliminary study certainly suggest that the authority to prescribe provides a significant avenue by which psychologists can be viewed as full service providers in the primary health care field. The prescribing–medical psychologists interviewed in this study indicated that the authority to prescribe and the collaborative relationship with the primary care physicians led to more frequent, thorough, and meaningful interchanges with the physicians. They are obtaining more referrals from physicians. They are working more closely with physicians with more medically challenged, dually diagnosed patients. New opportunities are arising for them to obtain consulting positions in primary health care facilities, such as prisons and health clinics.

The pioneer prescribing–medical psychologists in private practice in New Mexico and Louisiana have been practicing for more than 5 years. Many thousands of prescriptions have been written without any documented significant, untoward events. Hopefully, future efficacy studies will verify the prescribing–medical psychologists to be safe and highly efficacious providers. At present, this survey study elucidates a number of important qualitative aspects of treatment of the prescribing–medical psychologists in private practice.

The prescribing–medical psychologists in private practice are maintaining a psychological orientation to their prescribing, integrating psychotherapy with medication management. Opponents to the prescriptive authority movement have been concerned that psychologists would eschew this orientation and adopt a more classic medical model of medication management. Consistently, the prescribing–medical psychologists in independent practice in Louisiana and New Mexico emphasized that maintaining a strong relationship with the patient has facilitated compliance. The prescribing–medical psychologists who were interviewed adopted an integrated model in which they continue to use their psychological skills as a primary tool.

However, as of yet the authority to prescribe has not significantly reduced the difficulty psychologists experience in dealing with insurance companies and managed care agencies. Although a number of insurance carriers are paying psychologists for medication management along with psychotherapy, they may not be doing so at a rate commensurate with psychiatrists. Thus, these initial studies indicate the need for more advocacy fighting for equity in fee reimbursement and privileges for psychologists with their medical colleagues. It is in the public interest to end any inequity in payments of psychologists and physicians for psychopharmacological services, especially because the combination of psychotherapy and medication management creates the potential for more thorough and less expensive care in the long run. We must continue bringing public and governmental attention to the lack of appropriate remuneration for psychologists, as we did in reversing Medicare–Medicaid cuts to reimbursement and equalizing coinsurance rates for mental and general health care through the Medicare Improvements for Patients and Providers Act of 2008.

Many of the prescribing–medical psychologists believe that they are developing and expanding the biopsychosocial approach to intervention with mental disorders. Because of the psychologists' collaborative and relationship-oriented approach to prescribing, the medication becomes integrated into therapy as a way of understanding patient behavior and building patients' autonomy and confidence in themselves. The evolution of this new model of care is an exciting aspect of the prescriptive authority movement. That prescribing–medical psychologists can prescribe safely and address the needs of many underserved populations is, of course, quite important. The evolution of a new paradigm in which the use of psychotropics takes its appropriate place in the overall treatment of emotional illnesses can be revolutionary.

Therefore, this preliminary study strongly supports efforts to continue passing state laws that grant appropriately trained psychologists the authority to prescribe. The ability to demonstrate our efficacy as well as to delineate the nature of a new model of treatment only awaits the licensing of a significant number of psychologists to substantiate the claims and hopes that are suggested in this initial study.

REFERENCES

LeVine, E., & Orabano Mantell, E. (2007). The integration of psychopharmacology and psychotherapy in PTSD treatment: A biopsychosocial model of care. In E. Carll (Ed.), *Trauma psychology: Issues in violence, disaster, health, and illness* (Vol. 2, pp. 282–311). Westport, CT: Praeger.

Shapiro, A. E., Dorken, H., Rodgers, D., & Wiggins, J. (1976). The legislative process. In H. Dorken (Ed.), *The professional psychologist today* (pp. 207–232). San Francisco, CA: Jossey-Bass.

Symm, B., Averitt, M., Forjuoh, S. N., & Preece, C. (2006). Effects of using free sample medications on the prescribing practices of family physicians. *Journal of the American Board of Family Medicine, 19*, 443–449. doi:10.3122/jabfm.19.5.443

9

PSYCHOLOGISTS IN PRIMARY CARE

ALAN R. GRUBER

Psychologists must think of themselves as health care providers and recognize that mental health care is but a subset of general health care. From the clinical, economic, political, health care policy, and other perspectives, psychology has incalculable contributions to make to general health care, but the profession has been slow to act on its own research findings that demonstrate psychological intervention reduces cost, improves quality of life, and increases functional longevity in large numbers of affected individuals (Barlow, 2004; Cummings, O'Donohue, & Ferguson, 2002). In this chapter, I discuss how pharmacotherapy is increasing the role of psychologists in primary care. First, I discuss the evolution of primary care, emphasizing that although primary care psychology introduced psychology to primary care, medical psychology integrated psychology within primary care. Then, I discuss several obstacles to medical psychology. Finally, I discuss the roles of medical psychologists.

EVOLUTION OF PRIMARY CARE

Over the years, medicine has invested a great deal of effort into defining what is meant by *primary care*. The modern conception of primary care can be traced to the Citizens' Commission on Graduate Medical Education, which was founded out of concern over the growing trend for physicians to pursue specialty practice (Mills, 1966). The commission report reemphasized the importance of general practice to the profession, and it defined the physician in general practice "as the primary medical resource and counselor to an individual or a family" (Mills, 1966, p. 37). The primary care physician (PCP) was identified as the individual responsible for maintaining continuity and comprehensiveness in care even when arranging hospitalizations or access to specialists.

In subsequent years the definition of primary care was refined further. Donaldson, Yordy, Lohr, and Vanselow (1996) provided an example of the current perception of what comprises primary care when they defined it as "the provision of integrated, accessible health care services by clinicians who are accountable for addressing a large majority of personal health care needs, developing a sustained partnership with patients, and practicing in the context of family and community" (p. 31; see also Institute of Medicine, 1978). This definition includes a number of key elements. Primary care should be easily accessed when the patient needs treatment; primary care facilities should be prepared to address a broad variety of conditions; there should be an ongoing relationship between patients and physician; the physician should understand the family and community context in which care is taking place; and the facility should be able to offer integrated care, meaning the capacity to address emotional and behavioral as well as the physical aspects of treatment. This model has been reaffirmed in the recent emphasis on the primary care practice as the "medical home," the locus for integrated and coordinated care across health care providers (http://www.acponline.org/advocacy/where_we_stand/medical_home/approve_jp.pdf).

Primary care is a term traditionally associated with medicine. The term *primary care physician* is used to refer generally to physicians who have completed residency training in family practice, internal medicine, or pediatrics, though obstetrics and gynecology are usually included as well. In recent years, though, other professions have attempted to broaden the field of primary care and carve a niche for themselves within it. Most notably, the doctor of nursing practice is intended to provide a foundation for nurses to become independent doctoral-level providers of primary care.

Primary Care Psychology

Primary care psychology represents one of the attempts to broaden the professional landscape of primary care. Primary care psychology is distinguished from other specialties in psychology by its focus on *integrated care* and *acute care*. From the perspective of the psychologist, integrated care is the comprehensive involvement of psychologists in the assessment and treatment of patients who present to primary care settings with conditions that involve emotional or behavioral components. Acute care means that the psychologist is relatively immediately available to intervene with the patient, much as would be the case for any primary care provider.

Psychologists clearly can make important contributions to integrated care. It has been estimated that as many as two thirds of patients seen by PCPs present with problems that involve emotional and behavioral components (Fries et al., 1993). Mental disorders, even at the subthreshold level, have a profound impact on level of functioning in primary care patients, and the bulk of mental health treatment in the United States is provided through primary care facilities (deGruy, 1996). For example, 60% to 80% of prescriptions for psychotropic medications come from PCPs (Beardsley, Gardocki, Larson, & Hidalgo, 1988; Mark, Levit, & Buck, 2009). This clearly is a population to whom psychologists, particularly psychologists with prescriptive authority, can offer valuable services.

An important watershed in the development of primary care psychology was the formation of a task force to explore the role of psychologists in primary care settings by the American Psychological Association (APA) Committee for the Advancement of Professional Psychology (1996). A number of authors have since justified the growth of primary care psychology on the grounds that health care and mental health care cannot be reasonably separated from each other (e.g., Frank, McDaniel, Bray, & Heldring, 2004; Gatchel & Oordt, 2003; Hunter, Goodie, Oordt, & Dobmeyer, 2009; Strosahl & Robinson, 2008). In fact, many psychologists can already be found working with patients in primary care settings (Frank et al., 2004).

Psychology has tremendous contributions to make to general health care, including reduced cost, improved quality of life, and increased functional longevity for large numbers of individuals (Barlow, 2004; Cummings, O'Donohue, & Ferguson, 2002). Unfortunately, to date primary care psychology has achieved at most a foothold in primary care settings. The emergence of medical psychology creates the potential for dramatically correcting this situation.

Medical Psychology

The term *medical psychology* has been used in a variety of ways over the years. Its first use was in relation to the application of psychological principles to specific medical conditions. For example, the University of Alabama at Birmingham offers a doctoral program in medical psychology that focuses on the assessment and treatment of medical and cognitive conditions.

More recently, Louisiana adopted it as the legal term for psychologists awarded prescriptive authority. This use of the term has also been recognized at the federal level by both the Drug Enforcement Agency and the Centers for Medicare & Medicaid Services.

The term has been used in yet a third context, one that integrates the two prior definitions in a way that potentially has important implications for the future of the field of psychology. In 2007, the Academy of Medical Psychology adopted the following definition for medical psychology: "awareness of and training in medical, psychological, and social factors that inform a broad spectrum of services including psychological diagnosis, treatment, consulting about the use of psychotropic medications, and prescribing of psychotropic medication within the scope of practice of the profession" (http://www. amphome.org, Mission Statement, para. 2). The competence to prescribe psychotropic medication is but a part of competence to practice medical psychology. Medical psychology combines primary care psychology with prescribing psychology in a manner that dramatically broadens the skill set offered by the psychologist in a way that is particularly relevant in the context of integrated primary care. Specifically, the medical psychologist can assess the emotional and behavioral components of medical disorders, and treat those components by using both psychosocial and pharmaceutical interventions.

OBSTACLES TO MEDICAL PSYCHOLOGY

Psychologists who are attempting to work in a primary care setting face a number of obstacles. One has to do with restrictions on the practice of psychologists as health care providers outside the context of traditional mental health. These restrictions in part reflect failures on the part of psychology itself. In the 1960s, the APA did not pursue inclusion in either Medicare or Medicaid. This decision has had long-term implications for psychologists' recognition as a health care discipline. Since then there have been some important victories, including the introduction of the Health and Behavior Assessment and Intervention procedure codes (http://www.apa.org/practice/cpt_2002.html) in 2002. For the first time, psychologists were recognized as providers of services to patients for medical conditions such as cancer, Alzheimer's disease, diabetes, or coronary artery disease. Nevertheless, the APA continues to struggle with the exclusion of psychologists as "physicians." As a result, psychologists are forbidden to bill using "evaluation and management" codes, which are restricted to physicians.

A second obstacle is psychologists' naiveté about medical practice. When psychologists are practicing in primary care, they enter the land of medicine. In that land, there is a recognizable culture and an accepted language. To practice effectively in that setting, psychologists need to become natives, that is, they need to know how to act and how to speak; they must demonstrate the basic knowledge that is common to all the others that inhabit the land. Some of this is relatively straightforward. For instance, psychologists who are venturing into medical territory need to be certain that they understand the medical acronyms that any primary care provider would know, such as CHF (congestive heart failure), CRI (chronic renal insufficiency), DVT (deep vein thrombosis), lap chole (laparascopic cholesystectomy; i.e., gallbladder resection), ASA (aspirin), APAP (acetaminophen), and so forth. They must also understand the hierarchy of authority and medical politics. Ignorance will mark them as an outsider and interfere with success.

For example, a colleague of mine was a senior psychologist who had never functioned in a general hospital setting before he was admitted to the staff at a local hospital. The first patient he was referred for consultation had been prescribed Colace, a simple laxative. The psychologist was unfamiliar with the medication and asked one of the nurses about it. That action was deadly. Soon, everyone knew about the new doctor who did not even know what Colace was. That simple incident dramatically slowed the process of acceptance by the staff, which in turn lowered the number of referrals he received. Whether it is fair or not, lack of familiarity with a well-known medication is perceived as a major lack of knowledge.

DeGruy (1996) summarized a number of other obstacles to medical psychology. Included in this list were patients who are unwilling to consider the possibility that a problem involves emotional components, or may even have a psychological cause; PCPs' lack of knowledge about psychological factors; economic pressures for brief office visits can interfere with patient disclosure; and the emphasis in medical education on somatic, biological, pathophysiologic processes and the implicit minimizing of psychosocial factors.

A final obstacle is potential resistance within the field. Psychology is unique among the health care professions in terms of its diversity. At times, two psychologists can have less in common with each other with a member of another profession. A clinical psychologist who is part of the emergency room staff in a hospital in many ways has much less in common with a psychologist working on human factors in aviation than with the physicians with whom he or she shares patients.

One unfortunate consequence of this diversity is that psychology has sometimes had a difficult time finding its voice. The failure in the 1960s to become part of Medicare and Medicaid occurred specifically because the leadership of APA at the time was concerned that getting involved in an insurance plan based on the "medical model" would ultimately change the nature of psychology for the worse. The struggles within the profession over prescriptive authority are not new; they have simply changed in form over time. One may expect a good deal of resistance to devoting less time in clinical training to traditional mental health conditions and more time to medical conditions.

Without appropriate training, though, psychologists are unprepared to enter into the primary care setting.

In fact, one goal of the emergence of medical psychology would be the psychologizing of medicine at the same time that the medicalizing of psychology is occurring. That is, the two would start to become more alike as both sides become comfortable with the biopsychosocial model of patient care. As Shah and Mountain (2007) noted, the medical model is about delivering interventions for health improvement based on the best available evidence; that is, the model of care should be based on what research suggests is best for the patient, not the values of one's profession.

ROLES OF MEDICAL PSYCHOLOGY

The roles of the psychologist vary across primary care settings, for a variety of reasons, depending on multiple factors. Blount (2003) distinguished among *coordinated, colocated,* or *integrated* collaborative care. Coordinated collaborative care refers to the interaction of primary care and behavioral health providers who are working in separate settings and seeing patients independently but maintaining communication about patients. Colocated care occurs when the providers work in the same location and often share staff and resources. Truly integrated care occurs when primary and behavioral health care providers work side by side, in the same shared space, using the same medical record and with an identified goal for the patient service.

Integrated care can itself take a variety of forms. This section outlines some aspects of the practice of medical psychology in a consultative relationship, in a hospital, or in a community setting.

Consultant

Anderson and Runyan (2005) adapted a table from an earlier work that described the interdisciplinary model of the Air Force Medical Service (Runyan, Fonseca, Meyer, Oordt, & Talcott, 2003). The table (reproduced here as Table 9.1) provides an excellent comparison of the general expectations that a primary health care provider would have for a behavioral health care consultant as opposed to a mental health specialist. The actual functions of the consulting psychologist can best be illustrated by reviewing the components of a typical consultation report (see Exhibit 9.1).

The roles of the health care team members in primary care are generally determined by the PCP. However, given that many if not most primary care patients present with problems that involve strong psychosocial components, there may be instances in which the line between consultation and case

TABLE 9.1
Key Differences Between Behavioral Health Consultation
and Specialty Mental Health

Dimension	Primary care behavioral health consultation	Specialty mental health care
Primary goals	Performs appropriate clinical assessments	Delivers primary treatment to resolve condition
	Supports primary care provider decision making	Coordinates with primary provider by phone
	Builds on primary care provider interventions	Teaches patient core self-management skills
	Teaches primary care provider core mental health skills	Manages more serious mental disorders over time as primary provider
	Educates patient in self-management Skills through exposure	
	Improves primary care provider–patient working relationship	
	Monitors, with primary care provider, at-risk patients	
	Manages chronic patients with primary care provider in primary provider role	
	Assists in team building	
Appointment structure	Limited to 1–3 visits in typical case	Session number variable, related to patient condition
	15–30 minute sessions	50-minute sessions
Intervention structure	Informal, revolves around primary care provider assessment and goals	Formal, requires intake assessment, treatment planning
	Less intensity; between-session Interval longer	Higher intensity, involving more concentrated care
	Relationship generally not primary focus	Relationship built to last over time
	Visits timed around primary care provider visits	Visit structure no related to medical visits
	Long-term follow-up rare, reserved For high-risk cases	Long-term follow-up encouraged for most clients
Intervention	Limited face-to-face contact	Face-to-face contact is primary treatment vehicle
	Uses patient education model as primary model	Education model ancillary
	Consultation is a technical resource to patient	Home practice linked back to treatment
	Emphasis is on home-based practice to promote change	Primary care provider rarely involved in visits with patient
	May involve primary care provider in visits with patient	

(*continues*)

TABLE 9.1

Key Differences Between Behavioral Health Consultation
and Specialty Mental Health   *(Continued)*

Dimension	Primary care behavioral health consultation	Specialty mental health care
Termination/ follow-up	Responsibility returned to primary care provider	Therapist remains person to return to if in need
	Primary care provider gives relapse prevention or mainte-nance treatment	Therapist provides any relapse prevention or maintenance treatment
Referral structure	Patient referred by primary care provider only	Patient self-refers or is referred by others
Primary information products	Consultation report goes to pri-mary care provider	Specialty treatment notes (i.e., intake or progress notes)
	Notes made in medical record only	Part of a separate mental health record with minimal notation to medical record

Note. From "A novel approach for mental health disease management: The Air Force Medical Service's interdisciplinary model" by C. N. Runyan, V. P. Fonseca, J. G. Meyer, M. S. Oordt, & G. Talcott, 2003, *Disease Management, 6,* pp. 179–188. Copyright 2003 by Mary Ann Liebert, Inc. Reprinted with permission.

EXHIBIT 9.1
Components of a Consultation Report

Chief complaint and referral:
Statement of who requested the consultation and the reasons for the request. The question, issue, and/or problem needs to be specified.

History of present illness:
Specification of the precursors to the patientís current illness. When was the patient last doing well? When was the onset of the difficulties, and how long have they been going on? Has there been prior intervention?

Past psychiatric history:
Has the patient ever been seen in the past for any type of mental health intervention? Has anyone ever prescribed a medication for the patient for emotional distress, sleep difficulties, lack of energy, or any similar problem? What medications? Why did they stop taking the medication or stop seeing the health care provider following them for these problems? Is there any past history of substance abuse? What are the details related to the above? Who were the service providers? Was the patient ever hospital-ized for any of these difficulties? If so, when and where?

Past medical history:
What diagnoses have been established to describe the patientís medical status? Has the patient ever had surgery? What are the medical conditions being actively followed?

Medications:
Name, dosage, frequency, and route of all medications, over-the-counter agents, vitamins, supplements, or homeopathic preparations.

Allergies:
Identification of all known drug allergies.

EXHIBIT 9.1
Components of a Consultation Report   *(Continued)*

Review of systems:
Inquiry about various body systems; constitutional, cardiovascular, respiratory, gastro-intestinal, musculoskeletal, etc., and, in the case of issues pertaining to emotional or behavioral problems, specific information pertaining to sleep, appetite, sexual function, headaches, lightheadedness, blackouts, auditory–visual–olfactory–somatic sensations, incontinence, motor function, memory and other associated factors.

Laboratory data:
Review of available relevant laboratory and imaging findings.

Social history:
Marital status, family support system details, occupational and educational history, legal entanglements, and any other factors that impact on the patient's capacity to deal with the medical problems. Identification of psychosocial stressors.

Examination:
Standard mental status examination, including details of the patient's appearance, level of consciousness and cooperation, orientation and cognition, speech, movement, thought process and content, mood and affect, insight, judgment, and other associated variables.

Formulation:
Concise statement of the findings and the consultant's assessment of how these findings relate to the question asked by the person who requested the consultation and the patient's condition.

Diagnosis:
Multiaxial assessment.

Plan:
The consultant's plans with respect to following the patient or actions that may be taken independent of the patient's attending physician or other requesting provider.

Recommendations:
Suggestions that are being made by the consultant for the patient's care. These may consist of recommendations about the use of psychiatric medications, other consultations, imaging or laboratory studies, and so forth. In some inpatient settings, the consultants are free to move ahead with measures that the consultant deems to be necessary. In others, the consultant is expected to limit their practice to recommendations.

supervision can become blurred. For instance, if the consultant were a cardiologist, at some point the patient is likely to become primarily the responsibility of the cardiologist rather than the PCP. For the psychologist this situation can be more complicated. As a nonphysician, the expectation may well be that the psychological consultant is an ancillary provider who is serving at the behest of the PCP. If a patient presents with hepatotoxicity and continues to use alcohol, though, is there a point at which the medical psychologist should have a primary rather than consultative role in the case? This possibility may prove more attractive to the PCP than one might expect. PCPs find it very time consuming to deal with the psychological needs of patients and the behavioral factors that complicate their medical conditions. Furthermore, PCPs have neither the time, skill, nor interest to deal with those matters. As a practical matter, anyone who practices in conjunction with PCPs knows that they often want one of two possible outcomes from the behavioral health consultation: tell them exactly what to do or take the patient off their hands.

It can be useful to think about the consulting medical psychologist within the framework of the traditional classification of health care delivery into primary, secondary, and tertiary levels. A psychologist practicing in a setting that provides for immediate, first contact with a patient in a primary care office, clinic, nursing home, short-term rehabilitation facility, and so forth, is providing a primary care service. The psychologist who is practicing in settings wherein the primary care provider refers the patient for specialized services, with the expectation that the psychologist will assume essentially independent care of the patient, is providing a service that would be classified as secondary care under this descriptive system. Historically, psychologists who are seeing patients at this level are providing services that have been described as *consultation-liaison*. Associated with this role is the expectation that psychologists will communicate with the PCP about the patient's status to assist the PCP to treat the patient more effectively, even while proceeding with independent care of the patient as necessitated by their condition. Finally, psychologists who are working in tertiary settings such as inpatient psychiatric hospitals rarely serve as consultants to primary care providers. The role expectations and functions of the consulting psychologist will vary, depending on how they fit into this system in the same way that the system will define the functions of the PCP and their referral patterns.

Notwithstanding the above, an important issue that needs to be considered is how the psychologist will be reimbursed for the services that are provided. Health insurance coverage rarely covers psychological services for the consultative services described in Table 9.1. Thus, although it is true that psychologists could fill a very important function in these settings, the realities of health care policies and insurance coverage make it unlikely that many psychologists will fill these roles in the near future. Therefore, one would expect that the most reasonable efforts of individual psychologists and organized psychology would be to focus on patient care at the secondary level but with increasing attention paid to integration into the primary health care setting.

Hospital Practice

Collaboration is obviously easiest in settings where people are co-located, and nowhere is this easier than in the inpatient general hospital setting. For various reasons, however, very few psychologists are to be found on the staffs of general hospitals. Regulatory or policy barriers often play a role here. Another issue is that many psychologists do not consider the possibility of expanding their practice to general hospital settings, perhaps because they are intimidated by the expectations that will be imposed on them in the acute inpatient environment. The truth is that, as noted previously, these perceived expectations are probably reasonably accurate, and the medical psychologist needs to invest the time and effort necessary to familiarize themselves with issues not part of traditional psychology education and training.

The active involvement of mental health practitioners in general hospitals usually involves consultation-liaison. Leigh (2008) stated that

> consultation-liaison (CL) psychiatry refers to the skills and knowledge utilized in evaluating and treating the emotional and behavioral conditions in patients who are referred from medical and surgical settings. Many such patients have comorbid psychiatric and medical conditions, and others have emotional and behavioral problems that result from the medical illness either directly or as a reaction to it and its treatment. (p. 3)

Though this definition refers specifically to psychiatry, it applies just as well to the psychologist.

To a substantial degree, the consultation-liaison model of primary care psychology is an excellent exemplar of the required dual focus of the practitioner and the dilemma that is confronted in a primary care setting. On one hand, the psychologist is working in partnership with other members of the patient care team to facilitate the patient's medical services and expedite the diagnostic and treatment functions. On the other hand, the psychologist is expected to form a helping relationship with the patient and serve as the intermediary between team and patient. These two roles can come into conflict. For instance, it is often the psychologist's job to determine whether a patient has the cognitive capacity to sign an informed consent for surgery. Consider the situation in which the surgeon believes that the procedure is absolutely necessary, but there are serious questions about the patient's ability to understand that which he or she is being asked (perhaps, instructed) to sign. How much more complicated does this become when there are no family members to call on to help with the decision?

Psychologists working in general hospital settings may found themselves having to work with a broad spectrum of patients. The patient may have difficulties participating in their care for a host of reasons, including delirium, anxiety, depression, or agitation; psychosis, intoxication, substance abuse, or dependence; suicide, cognitive dysfunction, chronic pain, adjustment to a new diagnosis, or medical event; and many others. Thus, the psychologist is required to possess a considerable breadth of knowledge about diagnostic conditions and their emotional and behavioral concomitants. Consider some of the following examples that are taken directly from actual practice of a general hospital consulting psychologist:

1. A 61-year-old woman with a long history of bipolar disorder is determined to have renal cell carcinoma and can no longer tolerate the lithium that has kept her stable for years. Her lithium was discontinued, and she has become hypomanic and psychotic.
2. A 24-year-old man comes into the emergency room with abdominal pain. He is diagnosed with acute appendicitis and is taken urgently to the operating room. He does not tell anyone that he uses 20 bags of heroin a day. He wakes up and is out of control.
3. A 68-year-old man falls down a flight of stairs, sustaining multiple fractures and a subdural hematoma. He lives alone, and no family is available. His cognitive impairment is substantial, but he has no insight into his difficulties. He wants to leave the hospital against medical advice.
4. A 44-year-old woman with chronic schizophrenia and multiple past psychiatric hospitalizations is admitted to the hospital with pneumonia. Her attending physician is concerned about the possibility of psychiatric decompensation.
5. A 56-year-old woman is refusing dialysis and has decided that she would prefer to die.
6. A 17-year-old man is admitted to the intensive care unit after an automobile accident and is now quadriplegic and depressed.
7. An 88-year-old woman is admitted to the hospital after being found unconscious at home. It appears that she lives alone, had been on the floor, and had been unable to summon help, for 3 days. She is acutely delirious.
8. A 46-year-old woman who is a recovered narcotic addict is admitted with a fractured hip and is in need of pain management.

As these examples demonstrated, establishing oneself as a meaningful contributor to patient care in the general hospital setting can be a challenging but enormously rewarding opportunity for psychologists. The capacity to expand practice and obtain increasing authority as health care professionals will be achieved with much greater facility if psychologists achieve greater visibility in the health care arena. Doing so requires significant investment in the acquisition of additional skills and qualifications.

Community–Outpatient Practice

As medical practitioners are faced with increasing pressure from insurance carriers to limit their time with patients, they are becoming increasingly vigilant about ways they can meet patient needs while still managing the volume of service they consider optimal to maintain their practice. Collaboration with psychologists provides one way that PCPs can achieve this balance.

Medical care has changed dramatically over the past decade. The average number of days that a patient spends in the hospital has declined significantly (DeFrances & Hall, 2007). In many hospitals PCPs no longer perform daily hospital rounds, instead deferring to the system of *hospitalist* (i.e., most typically, internal medicine specialists whose practices are devoted to inpatient medicine; generally, they do not maintain outpatient, community practices) care for their patients who need to be admitted. Thus, it is likely that the greatest opportunities for integration and coordination of the physical and mental health needs of patients will be found in office-based practice.

A number of excellent volumes have been published to assist psychologists with the details of establishing working relationships with medical care providers (e.g., Frank et al., 2007; Hunter et al., 2009). The two threads that persistently run through such discussions are accessibility and usefulness. That is, PCPs need to know that when they refer patients, patients are going to be seen on a timely basis, and the issues that have brought the patients to psychologists are going to be managed effectively enough to reduce the burden on the PCPs.

Thus, one of the most important tasks confronting psychologists is to demonstrate their skill to PCPs once that first referral occurs. The quality of the report sent to the PCP is the best form of advertising for clinicians who are attempting to establish a practice. As has been suggested previously, in the context of primary care a report will be judged in part on the basis of familiarity with the language of medicine, as well as the ability to communicate about details of the patient's condition that may impact on the patient's treatment. For instance, for patients with diabetes mellitus, it means that the psychologist needs to know about (a) how to control the disease, (b) what patients need to do to maintain their health in light of the disease, (c) what the implications are that are failing to control the disease, (d) what the implications are of diabetic ketoacidosis, and (e) a variety of other factors that impact on the care to be provided by the psychologist.

Working in outpatient settings has many advantages. There is less urgency than in the inpatient setting, allowing for a more comprehensive and directed approach to assessment and treatment. The outpatient setting is also associated with lower levels of stress and time pressure. Seeing a patient over a longer period of time, with less intensity, in an environment under the control of the practitioner, allows for a greater degree of privacy without the interruptions that are inevitable in the hospital setting. It also permits access to those family and community contextual factors that are thought to be at the heart of primary care.

For the psychologist who has achieved expertise in medical psychology, the outpatient setting offers major opportunities for practice growth and meaningful contribution to the community in which they practice. It allows the psychologist to use a broader set of skills that are often desperately needed by referring clinicians and patients. The partnerships that evolve within the local health care community serve everyone's best interests and serve to further establish psychologists as important and effective health care providers.

CONCLUSION

Psychology is at an important junction. It will be increasingly important for psychologists to invest the time necessary to develop a broadened scope of practice; otherwise, psychologists will never be able to distinguish themselves from nondoctoral professions that are providing psychotherapy. The future of psychological practice may be in question unless more psychologists confront this challenge.

Part of this challenge is rebranding psychology as health care—rather than as mental health care—providers. Psychologists can play an important role in addressing issues of compliance, motivation for recovery, behavioral and personality changes secondary to medications or disease processes, and so forth, that are an essential part of integrated primary care. The opportunities are there: Knowledgeable PCPs are requesting those services for their patients in increasing numbers. Individual psychologists and educational institutions will have to decide how the profession will respond.

REFERENCES

Anderson, B. R., & Runyan, C. N. (2005). A primer on the consultation model of primary care behavioral health integration. In L. C. James & R. A. Folen (Eds.), *The primary care consultant: The next frontier for psychologists in hospitals and clinics* (pp. 9–27). Washington, DC: American Psychological Association.

Barlow, D. H. (2004). Psychological treatments. *American Psychologist, 59,* 869–878. doi:10.1037/0003-066X.59.9.869

Beardsley, R. S., Gardocki, G. J., Larson, D. B., & Hidalgo, J. (1988). Prescribing of psychotropic medication by primary care physicians and psychiatrists. *Archives of General Psychiatry, 45,* 1117–1119.

Blount, A. (2003). Integrated primary care: Organizing the evidence. *Families, Systems, & Health, 21,* 121–133. doi:10.1037/1091-7527.21.2.121

Cummings, N. A., O'Donohue, W. T., & Ferguson, K. E. (Eds.). (2002). *The impact of medical cost offset on practice and research: Making it work for you: A report of the First Reno Conference on Medical Cost Offset.* Reno, NV: Context Press.

DeFrances, C. J., & Hall, M. J. (2007). *2005 National Hospital Discharge Survey. Advance data from vital and health statistics; no 385*. Hyattsville, MD: National Center for Health Statistics.

deGruy, F., III. (1996). Mental health care in the primary care setting. In M. S. Donaldson, K. D. Yordy, K. N. Lohr, & N. A. Vanselow (Eds.), *Primary care: America's health in a new era* (pp. 285–311). Washington, DC: National Academy Press.

Donaldson, M. S., Yordy, K. D., Lohr, K. N., & Vanselow, N. A. (1996). *Primary care: America's health in a new era*. Washington, DC: National Academy Press.

Frank, R. G., McDaniel, S. H., Bray, J. H., & Heldring, M. (2004). *Primary care psychology*. Washington, DC: American Psychological Association.

Fries, J. F., Koop, C. E., Beadle, C. E., Cooper, P. P., England, M. J., Greaves, R. F., . . . Wright, D. (1993). Reducing health care costs by reducing the need and demand for medical services: The Health Project Consortium. *New England Journal of Medicine, 329*, 321–325. doi:10.1056/NEJM199307293290506

Gatchel, R. J., & Oordt, M. S. (2003). *Clinical health psychology and primary care: Practical advice and clinical guidance for successful collaboration*. Washington, DC: American Psychological Association. doi:10.1037/10592-000

Hunter, L. H., Goodie, J. L., Oordt, M. S., & Dobmeyer, A. C. (2009). *Integrated behavioral health in primary care: Step-by-step guidance for assessment and intervention*. Washington, DC: American Psychological Association. doi:10.1037/11871-000

Institute of Medicine. (1978). *Primary care in medicine: A definition*. Washington, DC: National Academies Press.

Leigh, H. (2008). Evolution of consultation-liaison psychiatry and psychosomatic medicine. In H. Leigh & J. Streltzer (Eds.), *Handbook of consultation-liaison psychiatry* (pp. 3–11). New York, NY: Springer.

Mark, T. L., Levit, K. R., & Buck, J. A. (2009). Psychotropic drug prescriptions by medical specialty. *Psychiatric Services (Washington, DC), 60*, 1167. doi:10.1176/appi.ps.60.9.1167

Mills, J. S. (1966). *The graduate education of physicians: Report of the Citizens' Commission on Graduate Medical Education*. Chicago, IL: American Medical Association.

Runyan, C. N., Fonseca, V. P., Meyer, J. G., Oordt, M. S., & Talcott, G. W. (2003). A novel approach for mental health disease management: The Air Force Medical Service's interdisciplinary model. *Disease Management, 6*, 179–188. doi:10.1089/109350703322425527

Shah, P., & Mountain, D. (2007). The medical model is dead—long live the medical model. *The British Journal of Psychiatry, 191*, 375–377. doi:10.1192/bjp.bp.107.037242

Strosahl, K., & Robinson, P. (2008). The primary care behavioral health model: Applications to prevention, acute care and chronic condition management. In R. Keesler & D. Stafford (Eds.), *Collaborative medicine case studies: Evidence in practice* (pp. 85–95). New York, NY: Springer. doi:10.1007/978-0-387-76894-6_8

10

PRESCRIBING FOR SCHOOL-AGED PATIENTS

BRUCE K. McCORMICK

Treatment of childhood mental disorders with psychotropic medication is becoming increasingly frequent as research finds biological etiologies or sequelae for many disorders of mood, behavior, or academic performance once attributed to faulty parenting, poor motivation, or flawed characterological development (I. Costello, Wong, & Nunn, 2004). In years past, psychologists have been called on for diagnosis of mental disorders and to provide psychotherapy as well as recommendations for pharmacological treatments. As we have moved into the 21st century, applied psychology has advanced to include prescriptive authority. Prescribing psychologists are now able to provide a comprehensive level of care in which principles of child development, cognitive functioning, and mental health are directly integrated with the technology of psychopharmacology. In the years since the first prescription was written by a psychologist in the United States, prescribing psychology has expanded, and the lay public and professional community are growing increasingly aware of its existence and value.

Prescribing by psychologists is still a relatively new enterprise, however, and there are only a few who are delivering services to patients of school age. This chapter is based on the author's experiences in the transition from a traditional pediatric psychological practice to one that includes pharmacotherapy.

It is not in any way intended to be definitive, comprehensive, or uniquely authoritative. Rather, its purpose is simply to offer some tips that have been found useful and to stimulate discussion of issues in the integration of traditional psychological health care with medication management for school-aged patients. Occasional reference is made to specific medications when doing so may clarify a point of discussion, but no attempt is made to provide a guide for matching available medications with currently recognized behavioral health conditions. Given the rapidity with which advances are made in psychopharmacology, our understanding of human genetics, and pediatric psychopathology, supplementing existing references with journals and continuing education programs is probably the most efficient way to maintain an up-to-date knowledge base.

ISSUES TO CONSIDER WHEN WORKING WITH CHILDREN

Psychologists who work with children must stay mindful that cognitive development affects symptom presentation just as physical development produces variable and dynamic pharmacokinetics. Pediatric patients are biologically complex, developmentally dynamic, and psychosocially diverse. Their typical day is spent in performance-based situations in which conduct is monitored and cognitive efficacy is explicitly graded; one in which social comparison is constant and time constraints are designed for group compliance. Within that context are vast mental health needs that have been underestimated by epidemiologists and underdiagnosed by practitioners (E. J. Costello, Mustillo, Erkanli, Keeler, & Angold, 2003; Roberts, Attkisson, & Rosenblatt, 1998). Many conditions that require behavioral treatment first become evident during the school years. In some cases, signs of mood, anxiety, and developmental disorders do not emerge until first or second grade. Other times, anomalous behavior only becomes apparent when an experienced teacher sees it in comparison to others of the same age. Conditions that are typically associated with adult onset may become apparent during the high school years.

Information From School Personnel

Referral for psychological consultation often follows a school-based evaluation from a multidisciplinary team. Comprehensive data from individuals with a variety of allied health disciplines can be invaluable in forming diagnostic impressions. However, each discipline has its own focus and therefore potential for bias. Consequently, there will be times when input from several disciplines may be analogous to the ancient Indian proverb of six blind men examining an elephant: each accurate within the limits of its own experience but requiring integration of the collective input to gain a complete understanding. For example, an educational diagnostician may report a child to have a deficiency in reading comprehension, whereas the speech pathologist may note evidence of a central auditory processing disorder, and the occupational therapist may describe unusually poor handwriting and fine motor skills. The same child may be described by the school disciplinarian as impulsive and nonresponsive to consequences, whereas the teacher who focuses on classroom performance may describe him or her as off-task and inconsistent in the classroom. Indeed, each team member may suggest treatment activities designed to address each of these concerns, although such a conglomeration of treatment activities would likely be chaotic, overwhelming, and almost impossible to implement on a consistent basis. Moreover, each discipline-based evaluation by itself might not provide a very strong case for pharmacological treatment, yet this cluster of concerns would be completely consistent with and perhaps all accounted for by an overriding condition such as the combined type of attention-deficit/hyperactivity disorder (ADHD). It is incumbent on the prescribing psychologist to have not only a good working relationship with members of a multidisciplinary team but also an understanding of the areas of expertise that each offers so information can be properly integrated.

When a referral comes from the school setting, it is likely that academic problems are identified as a primary concern. In such cases, it is important to rule out physical, emotional, or both types of conditions that could mimic, exacerbate, or occur as a result of behavioral health problems. For example, although medication is not typically used to treat problems such as dyslexia, dysgraphia, or dyscalculia, such academic problems can result from concentration impaired by a mood or anxiety disorder. Subjective emotional distress often occurs as a primary cause of learning problems or as secondary to learning disorders. Consequently, prescribing psychologists who work with students need to be knowledgeable about or have a ready source of consultation with individuals who are familiar with age-appropriate academic performance and learning disorders.

Working With Parents

Among the most critical aspects of mental health treatment with children are the detailed and ongoing interactions with parents or caregivers. Some will readily welcome our assistance, but there will be others who would not independently seek psychological services for their children and do so, perhaps reluctantly, because a teacher or pediatrician has made the recommendation. This means that permission for and active participation in treatment must come from adults who would not necessarily choose or accept behavioral health services for themselves. As a result, their understanding of and comfort with mental health treatment tends to vary more than is true of the typical person who is seeking outpatient treatment. For many individuals who do not seek treatment for themselves, their main source of information about psychological services may have been the entertainment media or cultural folklore. Some will have an expectation that mental health treatment is all powerful; others may be skeptical or even fearful. Such apprehensions and misconceptions can become potentiated further when treatment includes psychotropic medications (McLeod, Pescosolido, Takeuchi, & Falkenberg, 2004). Indeed, it is quite common for parents to preface their initial description of the presenting concern with a remark such as, "I don't want to put my child on any medication, but she (or he) is having trouble with . . ." Consequently, while all psychologists who work with children recognize the importance of ensuring that parents' concerns are heard, it is particularly important for the prescribing psychologist to enlist parents as allies in treatment. Whatever their initial level of comfort in seeking psychological assistance, information from parents is essential in evaluating the need for treatment and in developing a treatment plan. Their cooperation is a necessary part of medical management, and they have the right to decline or terminate any course of treatment. Much of the job of the prescribing psychologist will involve providing information about the use of medications in a way that is respectful, understandable, and that allows parents to understand what medications can and cannot do and why they might be beneficial for a given child. Our therapeutic training and the time and effort we invest in listening to parents, including them in the selection of treatment options, and providing them with information about behavioral emotional disorders, set prescribing psychologists apart from prescribers who have a more traditional, biological background. In so doing, we may realize an advantage in gaining relevant diagnostic information, promoting treatment compliance, and receiving ongoing reports about tolerance and efficacy of medications prescribed. Additionally, as their previous experience with prescribers will have most likely been in the context of primary medical care, it may be necessary to explain the nature and frequency of visits for combined psychosocial and pharmacological treatment. The key point is this: If medical psychologists remember that we are first and foremost psychologists, and if we use our skills to full advantage, we can radically improve the quality of medication management over other professions trained in a more traditional medical model.

Those of us who work with children know that sometimes parents or caregivers disagree about the nature and severity of their child's difficulties. Just as it is frequently the case that one parent believes the child needs only for the other parent to be a stronger disciplinarian, it is also common for caregivers to differ in their receptiveness to the use of medication. Disparate descriptions may indicate such differences. A parent who is apprehensive about medication may minimize the presenting issues, whereas one who believes medication would be of great benefit might describe the child's every flaw and foible. As with any psychological intervention, it is desirable to seek a mutually acceptable course of treatment; obviously, that goal is particularly important when a regimen includes the use of medication. Therefore, it is especially advantageous for the prescribing psychologist to interview all adult caregivers whenever possible and explore and attempt to resolve any differences in the concerns parents describe.

A situation all too often encountered is one in which inconsistency in a child's home life compromises the regularity of the administration of medicine. Such difficulty may occur when a single parent is too overwhelmed to provide adequate monitoring, or when a secondary caregiver such as a grandparent keeps a child for several days during the week. Perhaps most common, however, is the case in which divorced parents disagree about whether a child should be treated with medication and the child spends substantial time in each parent's home. It is not unusual to find a child who benefits greatly from medication and for whom one parent willingly follows the medical instructions while the other refuses to do so. Obviously, the most desirable course of action would be to find a treatment plan acceptable to both parents. When that cannot be accomplished, the prescribing psychologist may need to be particularly innovative. Sometimes arrangements can be made to have necessary medications administered by a school nurse, so that there is consistency at least on weekdays. That procedure may be particularly advantageous if the child spends alternate weeks in each parent's home. When weekend compliance may be uncertain, consideration of the pharmacological properties of specific medications can be useful. For instance, if a child takes a stimulant for ADHD, withholding the medication on weekends and school holidays may pose few problems—and may even be desirable. If the child needs a selective serotonin reuptake inhibitor, a medication such as fluoxetine may be preferred because the long half-life of the active metabolite may provide sufficient efficacy throughout a weekend visit. Even when it is known that there may be a difference in compliance with protocol between the parent's homes, it would seldom, if ever, be advisable to prescribe medication without the awareness of both parents. The prescribing psychologist needs to be knowledgeable of both ethical principles and state statutes in regard to parents' rights to request and refuse treatment.

When prescribing drugs that have abuse potential, it is wise to be mindful of the possibility of diversion (especially with stimulants). Particularly noteworthy are patients for whom refills of controlled substances are repeatedly requested exactly on or just before the expected date or when a parent requests a replacement of a prescription for controlled substance that has been lost. (One of the author's colleagues requires a written police report for a lost or stolen prescription before giving a replacement copy for scheduled drugs.) There can be situations in which reliable parents report that medication seems to have run out earlier than it should. In those circumstances, it may be worthwhile to discuss the possibility that friends (especially if the patient is a teen) or others such as family members, housekeepers, guests, or service personnel might have had access to the medicine cabinet.

Medical History

As prescribing psychology has become more widely known, we are often the first health care professionals to discuss the possibility of medication for a child, but currently it is quite common to learn in the initial session that the child is already receiving psychotropic medication from a psychiatrist or primary care physician (PCP). In many cases, they do not find treatment beneficial. One of the most important advantages of acquiring prescriptive authority is the authority to reduce or discontinue medications a child has been taking. Decisions to initiate, discontinue, or modify a medication regimen will be based in large part on information obtained from a medical history.

Prescribing psychologists who work with children should be accustomed to obtaining medical and developmental information, and the typical intake or initial interview usually includes questions about exposure to teratogens and other prenatal and perinatal problems as well as past physical trauma, infectious conditions, or systemic disorders. Many aspects of a medical history that psychologists traditionally would overlook or investigate minimally become important when medication may be part of a treatment plan. All current or past use of psychotropic medications should be queried as should any diagnostic work that might have been performed. We need to obtain as much information as possible about specific medications (to include botanical, herbal, or other so-called natural treatments) that have been used, doses, duration of each treatment episode, tolerance, response, reason for quitting or requesting a change, and any adverse effects. Also important is information about any psychosocial treatments concurrent with drug treatments. It is important to know whether there have been any injuries that compromised the central nervous system, long-term physical sequelae of illness or injury, or prolonged treatment that might have impacted attachment or socialization experiences or a history of chronic otitis media that could have delayed language acquisition.

It is also valuable to investigate sleep quality as chronic sleep deprivation from conditions such as primary insomnia or obstructive sleep apnea can produce inattentiveness, memory deficits, or emotional lability—conditions that could be mistaken for a primary mental health disorder. Additionally, sleep problems such as delayed onset latency, can result from emotional distur-bances and may give clues to issues that may warrant further investigation. Cardiovascular and metabolic history and risk factors should be explored in particular detail before considering medications such as psychostimulants or medications that could affect cardiac conductivity or weight gain.

Well-intentioned parents may still have difficulty providing medical information that is as precise and exact as would be desirable. Even when par-ents complete a written health history checklist, it is often advisable to dis-cuss their written responses during the oral interview, as doing so allows important points to be queried in more than one manner. It will happen, for example, that a parent will report a negative medical history but with more specific questioning will identify past episodes of loss of consciousness from a fall or prolonged hospitalization from illness. Similar skilled questioning is often necessary to fully explore family history of mental health concerns and response to psychotropic treatments. The results can provide valuable clues about possible genetic factors that suggest use or avoidance of particular phar-maceutical agents.

Consultation With Primary Care Physicians

A child's PCP should be informed of any medications prescribed both as a professional courtesy and to facilitate continuity of care. Even before decid-ing whether medication would be beneficial, it is usually wise to consult with the PCP as well as with any specialists that may be involved in a student's treat-ment. Doing so serves as an additional check for relevant medical information that the parents may have failed to report. Additionally, as a number of physi-cal conditions can mimic mental health disorders, it is important to know about a child's general health, and it is often wise to recommend an updated physical examination. Many medications require baseline laboratory testing. When the prescribing psychologist writes lab orders, it is often convenient for the patient as well as a professional courtesy to suggest the specimens be collected at the primary physician's office.

Standardized Assessment

When considering whether medication should be part of the treatment plan, data from actuarial instruments such as norm-referenced checklists and rating scales are useful in determining the extent to which identified concerns are occurring with a frequency, intensity, or both, that is excessive for a student's age and gender. They also serve to screen for comorbidity and for conditions that mimic, exacerbate, attenuate, or result from behavioral health problems. Many rating scales are narrow in scope and are essentially just symptom checklists.

Others cover a wide range of behaviors and facilitate cross comparisons because they are standardized with the same population for ratings by parents of both genders and by teachers. Two of the most psychometrically sound and frequently used of such instruments are the Behavior Assessment System for Children (BASC; Reynolds & Kamphaus, 2005) or the Child Behavior Checklist (CBCL; Achenbach & Rescorla, 2001). When using parent rating scales, it is preferable for each parent (or caregiver) to independently complete the same instrument. If that is not possible, then care should be taken to ensure that only one respondent complete the rating scales as they are not standardized for caregiver consensus. Parents usually understand the need for independent responses when it is explained that children often respond in different ways and do different things with each parent. Identification of areas in which parents agree or disagree gives clues to possible stimulus control or secondary gain for behaviors of concern and information about how the family system functions. These factors in turn can be the source of important hypotheses about the likelihood that each parent will accept and comply with the treatment regimen. They may also alert the prescriber to potential biases later on when parents are asked about behavioral changes that would indicate the need to continue, change, or discontinue medication.

Because children spend much of their time in an academic environment, it is possible that behavioral and emotional symptoms could result from problems with academic aptitude or a primary learning disorder. Genuine learning problems are not always readily apparent, and report card grades are of very little value in identifying such concerns, particularly in the early elementary years. Consequently, if there is any question about academic difficulty that is causing or resulting from emotional disorders, tests of scholastic aptitude and achievement should be considered. This may be as simple as reviewing the child's school record for past relevant testing data. Formal in vivo behavioral assessment, although often logistically difficult to accomplish, can be of great value in evaluating the effectiveness of medical intervention and in identifying possible side effects. Most school systems employ school psychologists who are capable of behavioral assessment, but their workload often precludes such a time-consuming activity. Alternatively, daily checklists can be designed for the teacher to complete. It is essential, however, to keep in mind that a teacher's time is limited and whenever possible to use procedures already in place such as daily behavior sheets or classroom internet postings.

If ADHD is suspected, continuous performance tests (CPTs) such as the Integrated Visual-Auditory Plus (Sanford & Turner, 2000) or Test of Variables of Attention (Leark, Greenberg, Kindschi, Dupuy, & Hughes, 2007) are often part of an initial assessment. Although they are sometimes regarded as if they were the gold standard for diagnosis, CPTs are subject to false positive and particularly false negative results (Preston, Fennell, & Bussing, 2005). Even though they are not absolutely definitive for ADHD—no single test is—CPTs are the most accurate standardized behavioral measures currently available, and they may be of particular value to the prescribing psychologist because they are sensitive to the effects of stimulant medication and can be quite useful in evaluating the efficacy of pharmacological treatment.

PRESCRIPTIVE PRACTICE WITH CHILDREN

A multitude of considerations are necessary when medication is to be part of a student's treatment plan. The prescribing psychologist must be simultaneously mindful of the conditions to be treated and how the child and the parents feel about mental health services in general and medication specifically. Potential misunderstandings will have to be anticipated and proactively addressed, and obstacles to compliance will need to be recognized and mitigated. Selection of a specific medication also requires mindfulness of safety and efficacy. Side effects may preclude the use of certain medications, such as those associated with significant weight gain for an obese or prediabetic patient. Yet the same side effect may be beneficial if the child is experiencing severely reduced appetite from concurrent use of a stimulant. There will be times when the mental health history of family members is useful in selecting medications. For example, a significant number of children diagnosed with unipolar depression will eventually have a diagnosis of bipolar disorder (Geller, Zimerman, Williams, Bolhofner, & Craney, 2001). Knowing that such a condition exists in close family members may suggest use of a drug that has demonstrated efficacy in treating depression and mood stabilization rather than an antidepressant that could activate excessive mood.

Off-Label Prescribing and Polypharmacy

Off-label prescribing, which is use of a medication for a condition or with a patient of an age for which approval has not been received by the Food and Drug Administration (FDA), usually occurs when there is a pharmacological rationale or some data that suggests a possible benefit but insufficient research to establish a medication's efficacy or safety. The studies necessary for the FDA to approve drugs for children are expensive and time consuming, and pharmaceutical companies have not always chosen to make the necessary investments to gain pediatric indications. Despite attempts by the FDA to offer financial incentives for testing medications with pediatric populations and a recent increase in consumer demand for drug research with children (Nature Neuroscience, 2008; Spiesel, 2008) there is still a vast gap between knowledge and need.

Despite advances in our understanding of child and adolescent psychopathology and an increasing array of available pharmaceuticals, treatment situations will arise wherein the presenting concerns do not match existing diagnostic categories, there are no clear guidelines for medication selection or for when the approved medical regimen is found to be ineffective.

In situations in which there is an abundance of information in support of off-label use of, for example, risperidone (Croonenberghs, Fegert, Findling, De Smedt, & Van Dongen, 2005; Masi, Cosenza, & Brovedani, 2001; see also Stahl, 2009), or when known mechanisms of action make logical medical sense, some prescribers opt to use a combination of medications (polypharmacy) or prescribe off-label. Obviously, such decisions require a conscientious risk–benefit assessment and a clear, balanced discussion with the child's caregivers. The American Academy of Child and Adolescent Psychiatry (2009) recently published formal guidelines for the use of psychotropic medication with children.

Black Box Warnings

Black box warnings are a mechanism used by the FDA to alert prescribers to potential safety issues with specific medications. One should never be cavalier about safety issues, and black box warnings clearly warrant serious consideration. However, the warnings are sometimes based on preliminary and inconclusive data and can be misleading, as was found for the recent warning about the use of antidepressants with teens (Gibbons et al., 2007; Gibbons & Mann, 2009). The prescriber must evaluate the relevance of such warnings for any specific patient. Indeed, any exception to FDA indications should be made with a solid understanding of pediatric pharmacology and the pharmacodynamics and pharmacokinetics of the medicines being considered. Any such decision should also be made following a risk–benefit analysis that takes into account the individual child's needs and characteristics and other possible pharmacological or psychosocial treatment options. As with off-label prescribing, any risk factors should be discussed with the caregivers and, when developmentally appropriate, with the child.

Efficacy

Diligent monitoring of response to medications is particularly necessary for children, as individual differences combined with developmental differences in pharmacokinetics and pharmacodynamics make the choice and dosing of medications particularly complex. For example, a commonly prescribed stimulant is marketed as reaching peak plasma levels at about 7 hr, although actual peak levels may occur anywhere from 3 to 11 hr after administering a single dose (Biederman et al., 2007; McGough et al., 2003). General guidelines are available from the FDA and other sources, but the biological complexities of children and teens require that dosing be done cautiously and on an individual basis.

In effect, medication monitoring is an application of a single-case experimental design (Barlow & Herson, 1984; see also Rizvi & Nock, 2008; Tervo, Estrem, Bryson-Brockmann, & Symons, 2003). Subjective reports from the student and anecdotal reports from parents and teachers should be supplemented whenever possible with more objective data. A number of instruments have been developed for monitoring side effects. It should be noted that comprehensive norm-referenced rating scales such as the CBCL or BASC tend to reflect typical behavior over extended time periods. For that reason, they are valuable for diagnosis but often lack the sensitivity necessary for monitoring the more subtle changes from medication over a period of days or a few weeks. Shorter checklists or symptom rating scales are usually more likely to identify improvements in behavior or mood that occur during the initial days and early weeks of treatment. Typically, symptom rating scales are short checklists of the most sensitive measures of behavior change that take place over the course of a few days or weeks. The BASC-Monitor (Kamphaus & Reynolds, 2003) is an instrument that has been designed to complement the more extensive BASC diagnostic scales and yet be sensitive to short-term behavior change. When possible, consider using data sources that already exist, such as classroom conduct reports.

When a prominent feature of the disorder being treated includes off-task, impulsive, or otherwise disruptive behaviors, medication efficacy is often judged by the amount of reduction of those problematic behaviors. A meager but intriguing body of research has suggested that for some children cognitive efficiency may maximize at a different (usually lower) dose than does problematic behavior (Sprague & Sleator, 1976). Although certainly not definitive, that observation underscores the importance of evaluating improved or declined academic performance as part of overall monitoring.

Prescribing guidelines for specific medications typically identify laboratory tests that should be taken at baseline and at periodic follow-up. Such monitoring is particularly important for medications that can cause blood dyscrasias or changes in liver function or that affect cardiac conductivity. It should be remembered that as children grow, physiological changes such as reduced relative hepatic efficiency can alter the effects of medications and regular schedules of testing should be observed.

Changes in appetite are common side effects of many of the medications used to treat school-age children. Antipsychotics and mood-stabilizing agents, for example, are often associated with increased appetite and weight gain, which are risk factors for obesity and diabetes. Some medicines, stimulants in particular, commonly produce appetite suppression. Indeed, early research suggested that with extended use, dextroamphetamine and methylphenidate may suppress normal growth. Subsequent research has suggested that although the associated appetite suppression can slow weight gain or even initial weight loss, those effects are usually transient and can be well controlled with prudent nutritional management. As a compensatory measure, clinicians have found that many children respond well to nightly milkshakes made with a mixture of ice cream and the nutritional supplement, PediSure. Regular monitoring of height and weight should be part of ongoing medication monitoring. Pediatric growth charts can be downloaded from the website of the National Center for Health Statistics (http://www.cdc.gov/nchs/about/major/nhanes/growthcharts/clinical_charts.htm).

Many medications require monitoring of cardiovascular functioning. Baseline and follow-up electrocardiograms (EKGs) are indicated for medications that can alter QTc interval, such as tricyclic antidepressants, many antipsychotics and mood stabilizing agents, and atomoxetine. For school-aged patients, monitoring of blood pressure and heart rate can be accomplished during medication checks or at the beginning of psychotherapy sessions. Recently, the American Heart Association published a position statement that recommends an across-the-board baseline EKG before starting stimulants (Gutgesell et al., 1999). The American Academy of Pediatrics questioned that position, and both organizations subsequently published joint guidelines for evaluating family history and risk factors in deciding whether an EKG or other baseline testing should be conducted (Perrin, Friedman, & Knilans, 2008).

Facilitating Compliance

Obviously, no prescription will be effective if the patient stops taking it. In general, patients often do not fill prescriptions or they unilaterally stop taking medicine. Discontinuation rates are particularly high for psychotropic medications and for pediatric patients (I. Costello et al., 2004; Hack & Chow, 2001). Despite an increasing recognition that biological factors are involved in many mental disorders and that medication can be an effective component of an overall treatment plan, within the general population there is a great deal of apprehension and resistance to psychotropic medications. Parents may need to be reassured that, contrary to popular belief, properly managed psychotropic medication does not promote but may actually reduce the risk of substance abuse (Wilens, Faraone, Biederman, & Gunawardene, 2003). This is a particular concern for parents with children who are taking psychostimulants. Misconceptions about psychotropics abound, including fears that the medication permanently changes the child's basic personality, eliminates volition, or renders them semistuporous (McLeod et al., 2004). It is often advisable to start medication on a weekend or during a school holiday so parents can closely observe their child. This can help allay some of the fears.

One of the most effective ways to promote compliance with medication is to spend as much time as is needed in providing information to the caregivers and to the child. It is essential that they understand why medication has been recommended and how any troublesome side effects will be managed. Providing detailed information, demonstrating openness to questions, and fully inquiring about patient or parent concerns initially and during follow-up sessions will do much to reassure patients and parents. It is a good idea to warn parents that information from the Internet is sometimes inaccurate or even deliberately biased. It may be helpful to provide some trusted, authoritative websites to parents who wish to read more about a medication or treatment.

Be sensitive to and inquire about cultural or religious factors that may produce resistance (see Pescosolido, 2007), and consider warning parents to expect well-intentioned but unsolicited and possibly ill-informed advice from friends and relatives. Recognize that no matter how great the need, a recommendation for medication is something parents usually hope will not happen. Emphasize progress and improvement when it occurs, and frame medication as a vehicle for improved functioning rather than a daily reminder that the child has a problem.

It is important to discuss with parents and caregivers available options that may attenuate discomfort associated with medications. For example, in addition to explaining that akathisia is a possible side effect of a given medication, provide a prescription for benztropine, and if the family has limited choice in pharmacies because of rural residence or insurance restrictions, suggest that the parent ensure their pharmacy has that medication in stock so if it is needed the prescription can be filled without delay.

Special Issues With Teenagers

Treating teenage patients can be particularly challenging. This age group is the most acutely aware of social stigma associated with and the most resistant to the use of psychotropic medications (Pescosolido, Perry, Martin, McLeod, & Jensen, 2007; Sirey et al., 2001). Often they will want to discontinue medications even when they have been stable and well-managed for years. It is essential that these students know their desires are heard and understood. Many teens appreciate being explicitly assured they are part of the "treatment team." It may be necessary to remind parents that assent from the teen is essential for effective medical management as forcing one to consistently take medication against their will is virtually impossible, ethically questionable, and therapeutically counterproductive. One practical approach with resistant teens is to discuss potential benefits of medication (e.g., less time required studying, greater control of their mood or temper, improved efficacy of concurrent behavioral interventions) and engage them in identifying outcomes that would indicate whether a subsequent trial of medication had been helpful. When a teenager agrees to which behavioral indices will be evaluated, he or she is not only cooperating with a systematic trial of medication efficacy but also effectively agreeing to the goals for therapy. It is interesting to note that some teens find alternative routes of administration—for example, a transdermal methylphenidate patch—less stigmatizing and more acceptable. Current guidelines from the American Academy of Pediatrics (1995, 2007) and the American Academy of Child and Adolescent Psychiatry (2009) include considerations for patient agreement to the use of medications. The teen years are often associated with experimentation with steroids, alcohol, and illicit substances. The skilled prescribing psychologist needs to maintain a rapport sufficient enough to ensure open and honest discussion of substance use when it happens. When a young child is treated for a chronic condition, it is not uncommon for a prescribing psychologist to follow that patient from elementary grades through high school and sometimes into their college years. We need to keep in mind that at some point our formerly young patients will go through puberty and are likely to become sexually active. Seventeen years is the modal age for initial intercourse among girls in the United States, and the United States has one of the highest rates of unintended teen pregnancy among Western countries (Meschke, Bartholomae, & Zentall, 2004). As many of the medications we prescribe are potentially dangerous to a developing fetus, we need to include frank discussions about sexual decisions, teratogenicity of medications, and proactive decision making with our female patients.

Difficulty With Oral Medication

Alternative routes of drug administration and alternative preparations may be needed to overcome another obstacle to compliance that is particularly common in younger patients: difficulty swallowing pills. Overcoming that problem may be a focus of therapy, and various training paradigms have been developed (e.g. Beck, Cataldo, Slifer, Pulbrook, & Guhman, 2005). In the short term, it may be necessary to select a medication that can be administered by transdermal absorption (e.g., clonidine, methylphenidate patch) or in liquid form. An oral solution of dextroamphetamine has recently become available in a strength designed for pediatric use. Other medications are available as an oral suspension (e.g., fluoxetine, risperidone). However, the concentration of such preparations is often stronger than desired for young patients, requiring dosing of less than one milliliter at which point accurate measurement can be difficult. In some cases, parents may be advised to measure and administer an oral suspension with an insulin syringe because of its small diameter. Parents may elect to have a pharmacy compound a medicine into an oral suspension, although that procedure can be costly, is seldom covered by insurance, and is usually only possible for short-acting preparations. Some medications can be mixed with water or juice (e.g., lisdexamfetamine) and tablets can often be crushed and mixed with applesauce or peanut butter, but parents should be warned against crushing or mixing time-release capsules that use a beaded release system.

CONCLUSION

Psychology is the science of behavior, and the focus of psychological treatment has always been the application of scientific principles to relieve suffering and bring about desired change. It is precisely that heritage of behavioral science that allows prescribing psychology to bring a qualitative improvement to mental health treatment. Having come into being outside of traditional medicine, the prescribing psychologist does not ask what medicines should be used; rather, which of the many tools of behavior change are appropriate for a given situation, and if medicine is one of those tools, how can its use be maximized by the concurrent application of psychotherapy and other relevant behavioral principles? The use of psychotropic medication with children demands diligence and care. The prescribing psychologist must consider all relevant data and communicate openly, directly, and frequently with students and caregivers.

REFERENCES

Achenbach, T. M., & Rescorla, L. A. (2001). *Manual for the ASEBA School-Age Forms & Profiles*. Burlington, VT: University of Vermont Research Center for Children, Youth, & Families.

American Academy of Child and Adolescent Psychiatry. (2009). Practice parameter on the use of psychotropic medication in children and adolescents. *Journal of the American Academy of Child and Adolescent Psychiatry, 48*, 961–973. doi:10.1097/CHI.0b013e3181ae0a08

American Academy of Pediatrics. (2007). AAP publications retired or reaffirmed, October 2006. *Pediatrics, 119*, 405. doi:10.1542/peds.2006-3222

American Academy of Pediatrics Committee on Bioethics. (1995). Informed consent, parental permission, and assent in pediatric practice. *Pediatrics, 95*, 314–317.

Barlow, D. H., & Herson, M. (1984). *Single case experimental designs: Strategies for studying behavior change* (2nd ed.). New York, NY: Pergamon.

Beck, M. H., Cataldo, M., Slifer, K. J., Pulbrook, V., & Guhman, J. K. (2005). Teaching children with attention deficit hyperactivity disorder (ADHD) and autistic disorder (AD) how to swallow pills. *Clinical Pediatrics, 44*, 515–526. doi:10.1177/000992280504400608

Biederman, J., Boellner, S. W., Childress, A. F., Lopez, S., & Krishnan, Y. Z. (2007). Lisdexamfetamine dimesylate and mixed amphetamine salts extended-release in children with ADHD: A double-blind, placebo-controlled, crossover analog classroom study. *Biological Psychiatry, 62*, 970–976. doi:10.1016/j.biopsych.2007.04.015

Costello, E. J., Mustillo, S., Erkanli, A., Keeler, G., & Angold, A. (2003). Prevalence and development of psychiatric disorders in childhood and adolescence. *Archives of General Psychiatry, 60*, 837–844. doi:10.1001/archpsyc.60.8.837

Costello, I., Wong, I. C. K., & Nunn, A. J. (2004). A literature review to identify interventions to improve the use of medicines in children. *Child: Care, Health and Development, 30*, 647–665. doi:10.1111/j.1365-2214.2004.00478.x

Croonenberghs, J., Fegert, J. M., Findling, R. L., De Smedt, G., & Van Dongen, S. (2005). Risperidone in children with disruptive behavior disorders and subaverage intelligence: A 1-year, open-label study of 504 patients. *Journal of the American Academy of Child & Adolescent Psychiatry, 44*, 64–72.

Geller, B., Zimerman, B., Williams, M., Bolhofner, K., & Craney, J. L. (2001). Bipolar disorder at prospective follow-up of adults who had prepubertal major depressive disorder. *The American Journal of Psychiatry, 158*, 125–127. doi:10.1176/appi.ajp.158.1.125

Gutgesell, H., Atkins, D., Barst, R., Buck, M., Franklin, W., Humes, R., . . . American Heart Association Staff. (1999). Cardiovascular monitoring of children and adolescents receiving psychotropic drugs: A statement for healthcare professionals from the Committee on Congenital Cardiac Defects, Council on Cardiovascular Disease in the Young, American Heart Association. *Circulation, 99*, 979–982.

Gibbons, R. D., Brown, C. H., Hur, K., Marcus, S. M., Bhaumik, D. K., Erkens, J. A., . . . Mann, J. J. (2007). Early evidence on the effects of regulators' suicidality warnings on SSRI prescriptions and suicide in children and adolescents. *The American Journal of Psychiatry, 164*, 1356–1363. doi:10.1176/appi.ajp.2007.07030454

Gibbons, R., & Mann, J. J. (2009). Proper studies of selective serotonin reuptake inhibitors are needed for youth with depression. *Canadian Medical Association Journal, 180*, 270–271. doi:10.1503/cmaj.081989

Hack, S., & Chow, B. (2001). Pediatric psychotropic medication compliance: A literature review and research-based suggestions for improving treatment compliance. *Journal of Child and Adolescent Psychopharmacology, 11*, 59–67. doi:10.1089/104454601750143465

Kamphaus, R. W., & Reynolds, C. R. (2003). *Behavioral Assessment System for Children-Monitor.* Thousand Oaks, CA: Sage.

Leark, R. A., Greenberg, L. K., Kindschi, C. L., Dupuy, T. R., & Hughes, S. J. (2007). *Test of variables of attention: Clinical manual.* Los Alamitos, CA: The TOVA Company.

Masi, G., Cosenza, A., Mucci, M., & Brovedani, P. (2001). Open trial of risperidone in 24 young children with pervasive developmental disorders. *Journal of the American Academy of Child & Adolescent Psychiatry, 40*, 1206–1214.

McGough, J. J., Biederman, J., Greenhill, L. L., McCracken, J. T., Spencer, T. J., Posner, K., . . . Swanson, J. M. (2003). Pharmacokinetics of SLI381 (Adderall XR), an extended-release formulation of Adderall. *Journal of the American Academy of Child and Adolescent Psychiatry, 42*, 684–691. doi:10.1097/01.CHI.0000046850.56865.CB

McLeod, J. D., Pescosolido, B. A., Takeuchi, D. T., & White, T. F. (2004). Public attitudes toward the use of psychiatric medications for children. *Journal of Health and Social Behavior, 45*, 53–67.

Meschke, L. L., Bartholomae, S., & Zentall, S. R. (2002). Adolescent sexuality and parent-adolescent processes: Promoting healthy teen choices. *Journal of Adolescent Health, 31*(Suppl. 6), 264–279.doi:10.1111/j.1741-3729.2000.00143.x

Nature Neuroscience. (2008, September 1) Credibility crisis in pediatric psychiatry. *Nature Neuroscience, 11*, 983. doi:10.1038/nn0908-983

Pescosolido, B. A. (2007). Culture, children, and mental health treatment. *Psychiatric Services (Washington, D.C.), 58*, 611–612. doi:10.1176/appi.ps.58.5.611

Pescosolido, B. A., Perry, B. L., Martin, J. K., McLeod, J. D., & Jensen, P. S. (2007). Stigmatizing attitudes and beliefs about treatment and psychiatric medications for children with mental illness. *Psychiatric Services (Washington, DC), 58*, 613–618. doi:10.1176/appi.ps.58.5.613

Perrin, J. M., Friedman, R. A., & Knilans, T. K. (2008). Cardiovascular monitoring and stimulant drugs for attention-deficit/hyperactivity disorder. *Pediatrics, 122*, 451–453. doi:10.1542/peds.2008-1573

Preston, A. S., Fennell, E. B., & Bussing, R. (2005). Utility of a CPT in diagnosing ADHD among a representative sample of high-risk children: A cautionary study. *Child Neuropsychology, 11*, 459–469. doi:10.1080/09297040591001067

Reynolds, C. R., & Kamphaus, R. W. (2005). *Behavioral Assessment System for Children* (2nd ed.). Upper Saddle River, NJ: Pearson.

Rizvi, S. L., & Nock, M. K. (2008). Single-case experimental designs for the evaluation of treatments for self-injurious and suicidal behavior. *Suicide & Life-Threatening Behavior, 38*, 498–510. doi:10.1521/suli.2008.38.5.498

Roberts, R. E., Attkisson, C. C., & Rosenblatt, A. (1998). Prevalence of psychopathology among children and adolescents. *The American Journal of Psychiatry, 155*, 715–725.

Sanford, J. A., & Turner, A. (2000). *Integrated Visual and Auditory Continuous Performance test manual*. Richmond, VA: Braintrain.

Sirey, J. A., Bruce, M. L., Alexopoulos, G. S., Perlick, D. A., Raue, P., Friedman, S. J., & Meyers, B. S. (2001). Perceived stigma as a predictor of treatment discontinuation in young and older outpatients with depression. *The American Journal of Psychiatry, 158*, 479–481. doi:10.1176/appi.ajp.158.3.479

Spiesel, S. (2008, October 15). Prozac on the playground: The dangers of off-label use of psychiatric medications in children. *Slate*. Retrieved from http://www.slate.com/id/2202338

Sprague, R., & Sleator, E. (1976). Drugs and dosages: implications for learning disabilities. In R. M. Knights & D. J. Bakker (Eds.), *The neuropsychology of learning disorders* (pp. 351–366). Baltimore, MD: University Park Press.

Stahl, S. (2009). *The prescriber's guide* (3rd ed.). San Diego, CA: Cambridge University Press.

Tervo, R. C., Estrem, T. L., Bryson-Brockmann, W., & Symons, F. J. (2003). Single-case experimental designs: Applications in developmental-behavioral pediatrics. *Journal of Developmental and Behavioral Pediatrics, 24*, 438–448. doi:10.1097/00004703-200312000-00007

Wilens, T. E., Faraone, S. V., Biederman, J., & Gunawardene, S. (2003). Does stimulant therapy of attention-deficit/hyperactivity disorder beget later substance abuse? A meta-analytic review of the literature. *Pediatrics, 111*, 179–185. doi:10.1542/peds.111.1.179

11

PRESCRIBING IN THE PUBLIC HEALTH SERVICE

KEVIN M. McGUINNESS AND MICHAEL R. TILUS

The prescriptive services of medical psychologists have benefited many people in many different settings. One of the most far-reaching organizations to integrate medical psychology is the Public Health Service (PHS), the primary division of the U.S. Department of Health and Human Services (HHS), whose mission is to protect, promote, and advance the health and safety of the nation. Within the PHS, the Commissioned Corps (hereafter referred to as the "Corps") is a cadre of more than 6,200 health care professionals who deliver public health promotion and disease prevention programs and work to advance public health science. The Corps includes officers from various professions, including psychologists. This chapter discusses the status of PHS psychologists in providing prescriptive services both inside and outside of the PHS.

CURRENT STATUS OF PSYCHOLOGISTS' PRESCRIBING IN THE PUBLIC HEALTH SERVICE

The majority of direct clinical services provided by the PHS are delivered by civilian and Corps personnel of the Indian Health Service (IHS) and Health Resources and Services Administration (HRSA). Each of these agencies is challenged to make quality health care accessible to its constituency. Below is a status report of the role that the medical psychologist who serves in federal agencies plays and a brief description of some of the challenges and successes that have been encountered.

Health Resources and Services Administration

The HRSA is the federal agency of the PHS that is specifically charged with increasing access to basic health care services for those who are medically underserved. The HRSA addresses access to health care largely through work with civilian health care practitioners. Within HRSA, many Commissioned Officers of the PHS serve in the Bureau of Clinician Recruitment and Service (BCRS). The mission of the BCRS is

> to improve the health of the Nation's underserved communities and vulnerable populations by coordinating the recruitment and retention of caring health professionals in the health care system and supporting communities' efforts to build more integrated and sustainable systems of care. (Department of Health and Human Services, n.d.-c, para. 1)

The BCRS supports HRSA grantees and other safety-net providers and health facilities by offering technical assistance and financial support of recruitment and retention programs in underserved communities, including various BCRS supported scholarship, loan repayment and recruitment programs, many of which are administered by the NHSC.

> Through the NHSC, clinicians serve in all 50 states, the District of Columbia, and every U.S. territory. Sixty percent of these physicians, dentists and nurses are in rural and frontier America, and 40 percent serve in inner cities. (The word "frontier" takes into account geographical and population factors. Generally, frontier areas pose greater access-to-care difficulties than do rural areas.) The 4 million patients treated annually by [NHSC] clinicians represent 11 percent of the estimated 36 million Americans living in areas that have little or no access to healthcare. (Department of Health and Human Services, n.d.-a, "National Health Service Corps," para. 1)

The Corps officers serving in the nation's underserved communities through the BCRS are called Ready Responders. Ready Responders are a small group of up to 80 Corps officers who, like other HRSA clinicians, dedicate their talents to delivering quality health care to underserved populations. As Corps officers and Ready Responders, they make an extra commitment to train and stand ready to respond to our nation's call in times of emergency. Like their DoD counterparts, PHS officers must have the capacity to relocate quickly and to practice their professions without seeking a license every time they deploy. However, unlike their DoD colleagues, PHS officers do not have preestablished posts or bases from which to operate. Nor do they have pre-defined patient populations in possession of active duty or military dependent identification cards. Rather, Ready Responders are most often assigned to federally funded community health or mental health centers (CHCs or CMHCs, respectively). CHCs and CMHCs, as their names suggest, are found within communities across the nation. Such communities are often co-located and well-integrated with impoverished rural or urban health professional shortage areas (HPSAs). Consequently, the PHS health care practitioner, particularly the relatively new medical psychologist, has a greater likelihood of encountering skeptical or uninformed individuals who may not understand their federal authority and may question the legality of their practice in a state wherein they are not licensed to practice.

The prescriptive authority of the first author (KMM) has been challenged on a number of occasions under such circumstances. Although the time consumed in resolving such disputes has varied from days to several months, the resolution has invariably been successful and involved the education of those unfamiliar with the scope of practice of medical psychologists and those unfamiliar with federal law and policy in relation to those of the States. When a Corps officer's right to practice medical psychology is challenged, the best tools are preparation, professionalism, and patience. In most cases, when provided concise, unambiguous information, cautious administrators will quickly recognize the right of the federal practitioner to practice without state interference. When there is resistance, it has often been because of fear of violating the law or losing federal funding. When the officer demonstrates a genuine desire to support the mission of the CHC or CMHC, resolution can come quite quickly. The same guidance applies to Corps officers who are serving in other community settings as are often found in the IHS, the agency of the PHS to which the majority of PHS Corps officers are currently assigned.

INDIAN HEALTH SERVICE

The IHS is the PHS agency that is tasked by the federal government with providing a comprehensive health care service delivery system for approximately 1.8 million of the nation's estimated 3.3 million American Indians and Alaska Natives. Members of the more than 569 federally recognized American Indian and Alaska Native tribes and their qualified descendants may be eligible to receive health care services provided by the IHS. A strategic goal within the IHS is to support the sovereignty of tribal governments in meeting the health needs of their particular service populations residing, primarily, on or near Native American reservations and in rural, isolated, or medically underserved regions. The vision of the IHS Behavioral Health Program is expressed as follows:

> To support the unique balance, resiliency, and strength of our American Indian and Alaska Native cultures, we at the Indian Health Service Division of Behavioral Health strive to support tribal and urban Native communities to eliminate behavioral health diseases and conditions; beyond elimination of these, the Division strives to promote health, resilience, and strength in all our communities. (Department of Health and Human Services, n.d.-b)

The PHS has a long and proud tradition of serving IHS service units (SUs) and tribally operated health care facilities. However, given that federally recognized tribes are sovereign governmental entities, it is often difficult to establish a prearranged and continuous means of information-sharing between IHS and independent tribal programs. Sovereign tribes have the option of hiring private practitioners or establishing a memorandum of understanding with the PHS for placement of Corps officers. Likewise, IHS SUs have the option of filling employment vacancies with federal civilians or PHS Corps officers. Thus, between the IHS and the tribal health programs there can be three personnel systems—the Civil Service, Commissioned Corps, and Tribal government—each with fairly distinct lines of communication and authority. Communication flow must, therefore, be based on voluntary cooperation and coordination from SU to SU and between IHS SUs, independent tribal programs, and interested partners. Although such an approach may work on a small scale, it is often difficult to collect adequate hiring data to monitor the state of medical psychology employment in tribal communities.

The precedent for psychologists prescribing within the IHS was set some time ago. Dr. Floyd Jennings (telephone conversation, March 18, 2009) informed the second author that in the mid-1980s he was prescribing at the IHS Santa Fe Indian Hospital as a "dependent privilege provider from a limited formulary." IHS responded to an urgent need for skilled psychologists and a growing demand for psychotropic interventions by permitting one psychologist, Jennings, to provide psychopharmacology and psychotherapy services. Of the 378 patients that he treated with psychotropic medication in the first year of his practice as a prescriber (under a collaborative physician arrangement) no adverse events were encountered (DeLeon, Folen, Jennings, Willis, & Wright, 1991).

Although all evidence may suggest that the patient care provided by Jennings to IHS beneficiaries was safe and effective, there were no licensing laws permitting such practice at that time. Even the New Mexico Psychological Association in 1988 recognized that there were no established professional standards for psychologist prescribers against which to form an opinion as to the ethics of such practice. That year, on December 9, 1988, a memorandum was released to IHS practitioners from the associate director, Office of IHS Health Programs, stating that

> in a limited number of SUs, clinical psychologists have been allowed by medical staff bylaws to prescribe psychotropic medications independent of physician supervision. . . . Therefore . . . I am hereby advising you that effective with the date of this letter, is it IHS policy that no psychologist may be permitted to prescribe medications independent of physician supervision. Operationally, this policy means at a minimum that any order for medication written for inpatients or outpatients by psychologists must be countersigned by a physician, preferably, a psychiatrist. (DeLeon et al., 1991, p. 257)

In effect, more than 20 years ago the IHS demonstrated that with or without physician supervision psychologists could responsibly prescribe. In the 1990s, psychologists in the IHS continued to make medication recommendations, often guiding the psychopharmacologic treatment of IHS patients. Such was the experience of the first author, who served with the IHS from 1994 to 2000 and as the chief of medical staff at the Acoma-Canoncito-Laguna Hospital at the Acoma Pueblo in New Mexico from 1998 to 2000.

In 2008, a request was made by the IHS for PHS mental health officers to be deployed to Rosebud, South Dakota, in response to a critical shortage of such practitioners during what has been described as an unprecedented suicide epidemic among members of the Lakota Sicangu tribe. It was within this context that the Rosebud Nation declared a national disaster and requested help from the PHS and the Aberdeen Area IHS.

Within HHS there are five disaster mental health response teams (MHT) composed entirely of PHS Commissioned Officers. The first author is the team leader of Disaster Mental Health Team Four (MHT4). Members of various MHTs, including MHT4, were deployed to support the Rosebud Tribe's request for federal assistance. In addition to support from social workers and clinical psychologists, a specific request was made of the MHTs for practitioners with prescriptive authority. As the prescriber deployed from MHT4 to support this mission, the first author became the first licensed medical psychologist to obtain prescription privileges independently in the IHS.

The IHS, from the perspective of the first author, faces many often daunting health care access problems. It also has a demonstrated willingness to consider reasonable solutions to health care access challenges without giving extraordinary weight to their popularity. Clearly, the IHS in New Mexico has provided a welcoming context to the concept of the psychologist as prescriber and health care leader in underserved communities. From 1988, when Jennings became the first IHS psychologist to prescribe, to 1998, when the first author was elected chief of medical staff for an IHS hospital, to 2008, when he became the first licensed medical psychologist to be granted prescriptive authority by the IHS, there has been continuous, incremental effort to improve access to mental health care services within the IHS. Whether during routine practice on the pueblos and reservations in the 1990s or the emergency responses of the 2000s, the psychologist in the IHS has been permitted to practice to the extent justified by training, experience, and law.

The use of PHS medical psychologists as emergency clinical responders can be seen as a naturally evolving effort to meet the need on Native American reservations and pueblos as the Corps strives to expand its emergency preparedness capability. Licensed medical psychologists are tangible personnel resources that increase the availability of comprehensive, quality mental health services. This is force multiplication "on the front lines" of rural mental health care, especially within Native American communities. This force multiplication is consistent with the PHS mission of protecting, promoting, and advancing the health and safety of our nation.

The second author was recently asked to research and lead a new strategic initiative to support prescriptive training and privileges among the psychologists serving in the Aberdeen Area IHS. Through the joint collaboration of the Aberdeen Area IHS director and the Aberdeen Area Division behavioral health director, a joint strategic plan was spearheaded in support of the clinical psychopharmacology training for seven IHS psychologists as a part of the overall 2007 behavioral health initiatives. The IHS Aberdeen Area behavioral health director, Vickie Claymore-Lahammer, joined this cohort and began formal training for prescriptive authority. Three members of the initial cohort were PHS Corps officers, and four were Native American civilian psychologists. The Aberdeen cohort's initial prescriptive training effort experienced delays and disappointments. Regrouping, the cohort found new resilience and support from the American Society for the Advancement of Pharmacotherapy (Division 55 of the American Psychological Association [APA]). Donations and incentives from private sources, the Irving and Dorothy Rom Family Foundation, the Psychologists in Public Service (Division 18 of the APA), the APA, and Alliant International University collaborated in a national collegial effort to see the Aberdeen Area Native American–PHS psychologist cohort become prescribing psychologists serving in Native American communities. Without the help of these national partners, the Aberdeen prescribing cohort's goal might never have gotten off the ground. There are currently six Aberdeen area psychologists in prescriptive-authority training now.

Facing often overwhelming mental health needs, lack of health care funding, poverty, extreme isolation with little infrastructure resources, hazardous weather, and high levels of alcohol and substance abuse, the Aberdeen Area Division of Behavioral Health director saw the potential mission impact of having psychologists in the small SUs who could also prescribe, monitor, and manage psychotropic medication. Recruiting psychiatrists to come to the upper prairies has been particularly challenging, and future prospects remain dismal. Almost all practicing psychiatrists that have been identified thus far have been located in the few, larger, settled towns of the upper prairies, far from the reservations. Many of the IHS SUs have also been unable to find sufficient numbers of candidates for their psychologist positions, given the shortage of medical psychologists. After hearing about the Aberdeen Area IHS's decision to support medical psychology, psychologists working in the Montana IHS region began their own quest for prescriptive authority. The Montana IHS region currently has four psychologists who have completed or are currently enrolled in prescriptive authority training. In a collaborative effort between these psychologists, the Area's chief medical officer, and behavioral health consultant, the group has recently developed and implemented a practicum and supervision plan to emulate the requirements of New Mexico's prescribing psychologists statute. A physician will be the primary supervisor on site at each SU, and a psychiatrist will provide teleconferencing consultation as an additional source of training and support. Several sites in the Montana Area IHS are also actively recruiting for prescribing psychologists.

Senior IHS psychologists and other behavioral health providers continue to offer guidance, support, and informed opinions on how the medical psychologist will be integrated into the IHS system at large. Among the many points that have been discussed with the authors, these appear to be the most current and germane:

- It is agreed that current laws and regulations permit state-licensed medical psychologists to practice in the PHS Commissioned Corps.
- Privileging remains a local process within the IHS SU, but a privileging pathway exists for the credentialed and certified medical psychologist.
- Collaborative efforts are underway to provide potential prescribers the appropriate medical practica and preceptorships within select IHS SUs, with the Montana IHS in particular developing options modeled after the New Mexico statute.
- There will likely be several PHS officers prescribing in the IHS within the next year specifically trained to provide service in Indian country.
- The PHS is actively recruiting mental health officers (in the hundreds), to include medical psychologists, clinical psychologists, psychiatrists, psychiatric nurse practitioners, and social workers.
- The IHS in several locations is actively recruiting for medical psychologists.

- Senior IHS psychologists and staffers have reported that medical psychology, as a specialty, has been generally accepted.
- IHS psychologists, human resources departments, and staffers are drafting new job descriptions for medical psychologists, which will be integrated into the federal grade–pay system, identifying the current and future duties of medical psychologists serving in the Commissioned Corps.
- Generally, the medical–clinical directors in the Aberdeen and Montana Area IHS have been very supportive of employing credentialed medical psychologists.

COMMISSIONED CORPS PSYCHOLOGISTS' PRESCRIBING OUTSIDE THE PHS

Department of Defense

Like the IHS, the U.S. Department of Defense (DoD) has played a pioneering role in the development of solutions to health care access problems in general and mental health care in particular. The role that the DoD filled in the development of the prescribing psychologist as a clinical resource in military settings was open, systematic, and objective. The DoD Psychopharmacology Demonstration Project (PDP; see Chapter 3, this volume) was begun in 1991 to systematically study the feasibility of training licensed clinical psychologists to prescribe psychotropic medications in the military. By 1997, the PDP had trained 10 military officers, who continued prescribing in their military assignments following completion of their training. As discussed in other chapters, four independent evaluations of the DoD PDP demonstrated that psychologists can be trained to safely and effectively prescribe medications and integrate pharmacotherapy into psychological practice. This preparatory work now supports another crucial solution to a critical shortage of mental health practitioners to serve our nation.

Over the past several years, members of the PHS and DoD have served together in war-torn countries across the globe. The vast majority of such uniformed personnel have been men and women of the DoD. To support our DoD servicemen and -women the "HHS is teaming up with DoD to increase the federal government's capacity to treat the mental health needs of our Nation's heroes," said Admiral Joxel Garcia, HHS Assistant Secretary of Health. "The healing of our injured soldiers, sailors, airmen, and marines is of top priority and the U.S. Public Health Service is honored to be a part of this program." To that end on June 4, 2008, it was announced that the DoD and PHS entered into a Memorandum of Agreement to establish an initiative titled, *DoD–PHS Partners in Mental Health: Supporting our Service Members and Their Families* (Department of Health and Human Services, n.d.-d).

Mental health officers in the Corps are now assigned to military medical treatment facilities across the United States to treat returning service members and their families. Some of the services that Corps officers will provide include counseling, family and group therapy, trauma rehabilitation, and psychiatric–medical psychology services for psychotropic medication management when necessary. In anticipation of this agreement with DoD, the Corps recently began recruiting more mental health service providers, including clinical psychologists, psychiatrists, medical psychologists, clinical social workers, psychiatric nurse practitioners, and other mental health care professionals. Given the DoD's 17 years of experience with prescribing clinical psychologists, it is not surprising that PHS medical psychologists have been welcomed under the new DoD–PHS partnership.

The individual Uniformed Services within the DoD have significant autonomy to establish policies and procedures for practitioner credential review and the granting of clinical privileges. Ultimately, military hospital commanders have authority over the privileging of individual officers. Policies that guide the privileging procedures for any particular DoD service are expected to guide the privileging process for PHS officers that are assigned to that service.

Prior to the DoD–PHS partnership, the Air Force and Navy had established policies for the privileging of medical psychologists. Air Force Instruction 44-119, dated September 24, 2007, Section 7.8.3.17 stated:

> Those clinical psychologists designated by the HQ USAF/SG, who participated in the DoD Psychopharmacology Demonstration Project (PDP) and were thereby granted prescriptive authority, may continue to have prescriptive authority for the remainder of their tenure with the AFMS. Prescriptive authority may also be granted to fully qualified psychologists who have completed a Master's Degree in clinical psychopharmacology, successfully passed the Psychopharmacology Exam for Psychologist (PEP), and who have received a minimum of one year of documented supervision. Supervision must be provided by a psychiatrist or a psychologist with prescriptive authority. (Secretary of the Air Force, 2007)

Navy BUMED Instruction 6320.66D, dated March 26, 2003, Appendix G, Clinical Privilege Sheets for Allied Health Specialist, Paragraph 6a, required that clinical psychologists who request authority to prescribe and dispense psychotropic and adjunctive medications must provide documentation verifying completion of the APA recommended training in psychopharmacology and successful passage of the Psychopharmacology Examination for Psychologists from the APA's College of Professional Psychology (Chief, Bureau of Medicine and Surgery, U.S. Navy, 2003).

On February 13, 2009, the U.S. Army issued a memorandum that clarified the policy permitting clinical psychologists with appropriate training to be privileged to prescribe medications for filling at the medical treatment facility (MTF) pharmacy. That memorandum stated:

> Clinical Psychologists who hold clinical privileges at an Army MTF may request privileges for prescribing psychotropic medications if they are a graduate of the Department of Defense Psychopharmacology Demonstration Project or meet all the following credentials requirements:
>
> a. A Masters Degree in psychopharmacology from a regionally accredited university.
>
> b. One year of clinical supervision by a board certified Psychiatrist or Psychologist with prescribing privileges in a Department of Defense (DoD) MTF. The year of supervision must include a breadth and depth of experience with a diverse patient population. . . .
>
> c. A passing score (70% correct) on the Psychopharmacology Examination for Psychologists administered by the American Psychological Association College of Professional Psychology. The examination must have been taken within 24 months of the time of initial application for prescribing privileges (United States Army Medical Command, 2009).

Although the DoD–PHS Partnership in Mental Health is new, DoD–PHS partnerships have existed for many years. The first author has served with his colleagues in the Navy, Air Force, Army, and Marine Corps during joint international health diplomacy missions at sea. The experience has, without exception, been a mutual learning experience that has been highly collaborative and productive. Many other joint-services operations have occurred over the years. The inclusion of clinical psychologists with prescriptive authority in the PHS and the DoD–PHS Partnership in Mental Health is expected to increase the demand for these health care practitioners throughout the DoD where their safety, quality and value is firmly established.

Department of Homeland Security

Division of Immigration Health Services

The Division of Immigration Health Services (DIHS) provides or arranges for health care services for undocumented migrants detained by U.S. Immigration and Customs Enforcement. On inquiry for this chapter Dr. Dennis Slate, DIHS chief, mental health services, informed the first author that he knew of no Commissioned Corps psychologists currently prescribing in the DIHS, but one psychologist is actively working toward a master of science in psychopharmacology from an accredited university. The DIHS acting director, Dr. Jeff Sherman, expressed his belief, in an e-mail message that as health professionals gain training and qualifications beyond the usual scope of practice, it behooves an organization to assess whether those extra skills and practice options enhance the mission of the organization. In the case of psychologists having prescriptive authority, Sherman expressed his opinion that such may enhance access to medical management of mental health concerns.

United States Coast Guard

The U.S. Coast Guard was a component of the U.S. Department of Transportation from 1967 to 2003, when it was transferred to the U.S. Department of Homeland Security. As indicated earlier, the Coast Guard is one of the seven Uniformed Services and one of the five Armed Forces of the United States. The health care provided for Coast Guard personnel is managed through the Coast Guard Office of Health Services, which manages

> healthcare to active duty and reserve members in support of Coast Guard missions, ensures the medical and dental readiness of all Coast Guard members to maintain ability for worldwide deployment, and ensures the availability of quality, cost effective healthcare for all eligible beneficiaries. (U.S. Coast Guard, 2008, para. 1)

The health care services for members of the Coast Guard are delivered exclusively by the health care practitioners of the PHS. Currently there is no Coast Guard policy to allow psychologists to prescribe, because currently the Coast Guard has no active duty psychologists.

Federal Bureau of Prisons

The Bureau's 35,000 employees are charged with ensuring the security of federal prisons, providing programs and services to inmates, and preparing prisoners for release (Federal Bureau of Prisons, n.d.). On inquiry to the Bureau of Prisons in preparation for this chapter, the first author was informed that, as yet, no psychologists have been privileged to prescribe medications in federal prisons.

CONCLUSION

The Commissioned Corps of the PHS is an agency for change in American public mental health. This view is provided through the lens of an expanding scope of practice for properly trained and licensed clinical psychologists with prescriptive authority. The PHS Corps is an essential component of the world's largest public health network. It is an integral part of the U.S. DHHS. Agencies in which Corps officers serve are many, however, the majority of clinical mental health services are provided through the IHS, HRSA, Federal Bureau of Prisons, and now through the DoD through their partnership.

Interest in the use of licensed medical psychologists as prescribers within these agencies and associated organizations appears to be growing, as is the availability of medical psychologists. The unique mission and distribution of PHS Corps officers across the nation yields quite a challenge for the profession and those charged to improve access to quality care for medically underserved communities. Today such "communities" include the impoverished, the isolated, American Indian tribes, members of the Uniformed Services, and the incarcerated.

The numbers of licensed medical psychologists and clinical psychologists in training for prescriptive authority is expanding. This bodes well for increased access to pharmacological treatments by those who would otherwise languish without proper treatment for serious mental illness. The PHS is actively using this health care resource. The public is benefiting and will increase its use of medical psychology so long as we, the practitioners, provide quality services and educate the public with patience and persistence.

REFERENCES

Chief, Bureau of Medicine and Surgery. (2003, March 26). *Bumed Instruction 6320.66D*. Retrieved from http://kentandassociates.biz/documents/Navy_Core_2003.pdf

DeLeon, P. H., Folen, R. A., Jennings, F. L., Willis, D. J., & Wright, R. H. (1991). The case for prescription privileges: A logical evolution of professional practice. *Journal of Clinical Child Psychology, 20*, 254–267. doi:10.1207/s15374424jccp2003_4

Department of Health and Human Services. (n.d.-a). *About HRSA: Fact sheets, clinician recruitment and service*. Retrieved from http://www.hrsa.gov/about/factsheets/bcrs.htm

Department of Health and Human Services. (n.d.-b). *Behavioral health announcements: What's new*. Retrieved from http://www.ihs.gov/MedicalPrograms/Behavioral

Department of Health and Human Services. (n.d.-c). *Health Resources and Services Administration, Bureau of Clinician Recruitment & Service*. Retrieved from http://www.hrsa.gov/bcrs

Department of Health and Human Services. (n.d.-d). *HHS, Department of Defense sign agreement to increase mental health services available to returning military service members*. Retrieved from http://www.usphs.gov/articles/dod.aspx

Federal Bureau of Prisons. (n.d.). *About the Bureau of Prisons*. Retrieved from http://www.bop.gov/about/index.jsp

Secretary of the Air Force. (2007). *Air Force Instruction 44-119*. Retrieved from http://www.e-publishing.af.mil/shared/media/epubs/AFI44-119.pdf

United States Army Medical Command. (2009, February 13). Memorandum for Commanders, MEDCOM Regional Medical Commands. Policy and Procedures for Credentialing and Privileging Clinical Psychologists to Prescribe Medications. Department of the Army.

United States Coast Guard. (2008). *Human Resources Office of Health Services (CG-112)*. Retrieved from http://www.uscg.mil/hq/cg1/cg112/default.asp

IV

LOOKING FORWARD

12

LESSONS FROM THE TRENCHES: GETTING LAWS PASSED

ROBERT E. McGRATH

No one is quite sure who first said it, what they actually said, or when or where the statement was made. It has been attributed to Otto von Bismarck, Benjamin Disraeli, Winston Churchill, Mark Twain, and various other less notable figures. Whatever the circumstances, it represents one of the great truisms about the legislative process: "Laws are like sausages—it is best not to see them being made."

I suspect few psychologists will ever have much to do with the sausage-making process, but achieving prescriptive authority requires a great deal of contact with the law-making process, and it is indeed not a pretty sight. Every now and then a dramatic event will facilitate the accelerated enactment of a bill: A child is abducted and within a week new child protection legislation has passed; the Patriot Act was approved in the wake of 9/11 even though many legislators did not know the specifics of the bill. These bills tend to get particular attention in the press because of their emotional pull and can distort one's view of how bills get passed. In fact, during every session of a state legislature as many as several thousand bills may be introduced. If there is no groundswell of support for a particular bill, getting it passed can be a slow and arduous task of building coalitions, shaking hands, making deals, accepting multiple defeats with equanimity, springing into action at a moment's notice, and knowing when to push and when to back off. It is a messy, nonlinear, and often arbitrary process. Psychologists who are trained as rationalists and ethicists, who tend to be a contemplative and an orderly lot, can find the process particularly alien.

At the same time, once psychologists understand the process of creating law, they can become quite effective at working with legislators. We tend to have better-than-average social skills, be adept at reading people, and come across as a dedicated and caring group. These are skills that smooth the process, but they are not sufficient to the task of getting legislation passed.

This chapter focuses on a series of principles I have drawn from my experiences working on prescriptive authority legislation for psychologists (RxP) in a number of states. These principles provide a rough outline of the steps required to achieve prescriptive authority, though they do not define a precise chronological system. They are also at times intentionally general. This is partly because they are intended to apply across legislative settings but also because it is not in the best interests of the profession to provide too much detail about the specifics in a public venue. For the more pacifistic of readers, I apologize for the references to a military campaign, but the metaphor applies surprisingly well to the legislative process in the face of fierce opposition. Achieving RxP has been and will continue to be a battle.

DON'T WAIT FOR THE GROUNDSWELL

Some state associations have been slow to get out of the RxP starting gate because they are afraid of getting too far out ahead of their membership on what is perceived as a controversial issue. My experience suggests that if you expect the membership as a whole to start calling for RxP, nothing will ever happen. For one thing, the typical member does not really consider the implications until the issue becomes salient. For example, it often has to be pointed out that supporting RxP does not mean that the psychologist is committing to becoming a prescriber. In polls about prescriptive authority, usually about two thirds of psychologists indicate they are supportive, but when state association members are asked to prioritize a list of goals, RxP usually emerges well below issues associated with our status as a midlevel or adjunctive provider, such as hospital privileges or reimbursement rates. This pattern suggests that respondents fail to recognize that prescriptive authority is our best option for enhancing our power in the health care system as a whole and will be essential to achieving the goals mentioned above.

Another reason for moving ahead is that support for prescriptive authority has always been driven by a small group of individuals who recognize the opportunities it will create. This was true when the American Psychological

Association (APA) first adopted RxP as a priority, and it has been true in every state with an active legislative effort. In fact, in most states it is possible to identify at most two to three people who have orchestrated the initiative. We can call them the "generals."

PICK YOUR GENERALS

The perfect general is rare. It would require someone interested if not already experienced in the legislative process, who will be a thick-skinned advocate for the cause, has good interpersonal and leadership skills, is adept at raising money, and is willing to commit 5 or more years to the process. In the absence of the perfect general, in most states a group of two to three people has emerged as the leaders of the movement, each of whom demonstrates at least one of the features listed. This division of responsibilities is also helpful as the generals provide support to each other through what is at times a grueling process.

Ultimately, the generals cannot do it alone and will need support from other members of the association and external consultants. Even so, it is important that everyone understands who is in charge. Legislative efforts require experienced leadership and a coherent message; they cannot be conducted as a democracy.

FORM YOUR CORE COALITION

The core players in the RxP initiative will be the generals, the state association, and the lobbyists. It is not always the case that the state association is the driving force behind prescriptive authority legislation. For example, in Louisiana the effort was largely spearheaded through an organization called the Louisiana Association of Medical Psychologists. Even so, the support of the state association is worth courting, though in some cases this step in itself may consume the first couple of years of the effort. Legislators are less likely to support RxP if the state association is clearly ambivalent or even skeptical about the bill. Furthermore, involvement of the state association creates the potential for state grants from both APA Division 55 (American Society for the Advancement of Pharmacotherapy) and the APA Committee for the Advancement of Professional Psychology. The latter in particular has played a major role in providing funding for certain components of the legislative effort.

Involvement of the state association also provides access to the association's lobbyist, although the advocates of RxP should seriously evaluate who is the best choice as chief lobbyist for the effort. RxP initiatives have met with fierce opposition from medical associations, and without an effective lobbyist the effort is probably doomed from the beginning. Among the characteristics of a good choice are a positive reputation in the state legislature (particularly with the party in the majority), prior experience with health care issues and perhaps even with similar bills, and enthusiasm for the goal. Over time it may be deemed useful to hire additional lobbyists, particularly if your chief lobbyist has a reputation of working more with one political party than the other or if the opposition blankets the legislature with multiple lobbyists. Unless problems develop with your first lobbyist, it is beneficial to have a lobbyist who works with you through the entire multiyear process.

PREPARE THE CAMPAIGN

Once the core group is identified, the next step involves preparation. Start by writing a draft bill. The lobbyist will be of assistance with this task. Many of the bills that have been submitted to date are available from the local generals. APA also provides a model bill (available at http://www.apapracticecentral. org/advocacy/authority/model-legislation.pdf). Unique elements of the legislative struggle may lead to various amendments to the bill; in fact, few controversial bills pass without amendment, and compromise is often necessary to get a bill passed. It is worth considering prior to submitting the bill which elements of the bill are open to compromise for the sake of increasing support and which should be protected. One particularly important example of the latter is C.(2) of the model bill. This keeps the training model and the definition of adequate preparation under the control of the profession.

At this point you want to have a good sense of the committees that will most likely hear and vote on the bill. You want to familiarize yourself with the unique qualities of your legislature. For example, in some states once a bill passes through all of the relevant committees its outcome on the floor of the legislature is essentially assured, whereas in others its fate is still uncertain. Committees and committee members differ in their influence on the ultimate outcome. It is unfortunate that the most influential members of the legislature on issues of health care are often nonpsychologist health care professionals who may be strongly opposed to enhancing psychology's scope of practice. You also want to know what role, if any, the licensing board plays in legislation for psychologists. In some states the licensing board plays no role, whereas in other states it is asked to submit an opinion.

Finally, crucial initial contacts are made. The lobbyist may recommend that he or she privately float the idea with a few legislators, or the lobbyist may organize some informal meetings with key legislators. The goal is to identify the sponsors for the bill, that is, the members of the state senate and assembly who will become its key advocates. Again, these sponsors should be chosen wisely. The degree to which the sponsors are respected by their colleagues is an important factor in the success of your bill.

TRAIN YOUR TROOPS

It is very important for psychologists in your state to receive the training for prescriptive authority. If you argue that RxP is important for increasing access, it is not uncommon for a legislator to ask how many psychologists are "good to go." Of course, the numbers trained will probably never be large until the bill is passed. You can point this fact out, but if only a handful of psychologists in the state have pursued the training, it makes the battle even more difficult.

Once committed to the training, those psychologists also become members of the coalition, the individuals who will help the generals sell the bill to legislators. It is recommended that the generals spend some time thinking about the strengths and weaknesses of the psychologists involved: Who are the good hand shakers? Who is the one to send in when the legislator wants the arguments?

In preparing these individuals for the struggle ahead, you have to walk a fine line between maintaining enthusiasm and being realistic. In several states I have seen a strong enthusiastic effort in the first year a bill was introduced, only to have the effort fall apart the very next year because the participants were convinced that they would win in the first year and lost hope when it did not come to fruition.

RAISE MONEY

I have avoided this topic for as long as possible, but it is time to talk money. War is not cheap, but psychologists are. We are notoriously poor at contributing to advocacy efforts. I suspect this unfortunate attribute reflects the low rate of reimbursement psychologists receive relative to the expense of training (a condition prescriptive authority may ultimately provide the basis for correcting). I also think it has something to do with those stylistic issues I mentioned earlier that result in resistance among psychologists to joining organizations and promotion themselves.

In fact, RxP can involve hundreds of thousands of dollars above any donations psychologists make as individuals to legislators' campaign funds. Good lobbyists, offering dinners and cocktail parties to present educational materials to legislators and their aides, bringing in experts from other states, professional-looking brochures, and regular trips to the state capitol are all expensive. Part of readying the troops requires letting them know they will be asked not only for time but for money.

It is important to know what the money you raise can and cannot be used to do. For example, some money that comes from APA may only be used for educational purposes and cannot go to supporting legislatures or lobbying. Violating these rules is unethical and dangerous; therefore, it is important to keep detailed and complete records of expenditures.

BUILD ALLIANCES

There are a number of groups with whom you want to make contact as you approach the point where the bill will be submitted. Even if the licensing board in psychology plays no formal role in the legislative process, it is probably appropriate to discuss the proposed legislation with the members, if only as a courtesy. Contact with consumer groups can be important. In several states, supportive consumer groups have played a significant role in advancing the bill. The largest consumer group in the field of mental health, the National Alliance on Mental Illness, is officially neutral on the issue of RxP, although local chapters have at times taken a stand one way or the other. It is worth exploring the potential for support from the local chapter.

In several states, local primary care associations have become important allies. These alliances have resulted from building a requirement in the bill for some sort of involvement in care to populations defined as underserved. This may for example involve service at a federally qualified health center or in a medically underserved area.

In a number of cases, advocates of RxP have approached physicians to solicit their support for the legislation. To my knowledge, no medical association has ever come out in support of RxP. Individual physicians have, and some have even testified in support of the bill or submitted letters of support, but more commonly physicians will indicate private support for psychologists' efforts but refuse to break with their colleagues. Similarly, we have had some luck getting individual nurse practitioners to speak in support of RxP, but nursing associations have not been generally supportive.

It is also worth making contact with the governor's office through your lobbyist. On a controversial bill, the governor is unlikely to formally commit to signing the bill unless it first passes the legislature. Even so, it is best to prepare for success and make sure the governor is at least willing to consider it.

TALK TO LEGISLATORS

Once the bill is submitted by the sponsor, things really start moving. In the coming months there will be numerous meetings. Unless the bill dies, each committee will have a hearing and vote on the bill. In between hearings, regular contact is made with legislators who are trying to get their support. Contact by residents of their district is very important. It is also important to make sure any questions they have about the bill are addressed.

I recommend warning the bill's sponsors that members of the legislature may receive letters from a small group of psychologists who are opposed to the bill. Point out that no change in a profession is ever achieved without some internal opposition and that surveys consistently demonstrate most psychologists are in support. Your sponsors will likely take this information in stride.

Interpersonal skills are important here. The legislator needs to set the pace of the meeting. Sometimes they are overwhelmed by their obligations and may want to know nothing more than the purpose of the bill and the name of the sponsor; at other times they may be open to a lengthy discussion. In particular, I have been surprised by how many are willing to share details of struggles in their own family with addiction or mental illness. If you believe the legislator may be open to it, do not hesitate to ask each to become a cosponsor of the bill. Increasing the number of sponsors will help build a critical mass of support. Being polite and respectful to both legislators and their staff is also essential.

In the last several years, Division 55 has become more active in state efforts to convince legislators to support RxP. In each of the last 2 years, members of the association who are experienced in lobbying for a bill have flown in and made the rounds of legislative offices with members of the local team. The combination of someone with expertise in answering even the toughest questions with someone who lives or works in the legislator's district and can discuss shortages in care provides a powerful one–two (punch).

Legislators often suggest negotiating with the medical society. It is for this reason that talks with the medical society early in the process are recommended even if not productive. This suggestion is best addressed by describing your efforts at such negotiation and the reasons for their failure.

HOLD LEGISLATIVE HEARINGS

At committee hearings, make sure you understand the rules that govern the proceedings, such as time limits and order of presentation. In particular, know whether you will have an opportunity to rebut points made by the opposition. Be respectful and nondefensive in response to questions or challenges.

Under the best of circumstances, if your efforts with legislators have been successful, the outcomes of legislative hearings have been determined before you enter the room. With controversial bills, this is often not achievable. If the votes are clearly not there to pass the committee, it may be worth requesting a delay in consideration of the bill while you try to garner more support. If it looks like the bill will not get the support it needs, you may decide to pull the bill rather than let a negative vote go on the record.

Whether or not the outcome is clear before you walk in the door, be as prepared as possible for each hearing. Make sure the person or persons representing your position are knowledgeable, level headed, and personable. In your testimony, you should be ready to present the case for RxP, and you should anticipate the arguments against. The opposition is almost guaranteed to focus on three arguments: psychologists are unsafe, anyone who wants to prescribe should go to medical school, and the shortage in care can be addressed through telepsychiatry. You can use the materials provided in Chapter 1 of this volume to help you prepare for the first two arguments. Those times when I have seen opponents raise telepsychiatry as a solution to access problems it has struck me as particularly dishonest, as a symbolic gesture that they take the access problem seriously. The practical problems of funding a telepsychiatry system, finding psychiatrists with the additional time to provide supervision, and leaving diagnosis in the hands of primary care physicians with inadequate training to the task are never mentioned. You should be ready to mention them.

BE READY FOR THE LONG HAUL

Getting a bill passed usually requires at least two committee votes in each house of the state legislature, a floor vote in each house, and approval by the governor or a veto override. It is a demanding, time-consuming process. The generals in particular will be spending many days in the capitol. There will be legislative dinners and meetings with various organizations. It can become a consuming activity for a while. Be ready for it.

BE FLEXIBLE

Each legislator may need a different approach: One may be concerned about over-medication and whether psychologists will follow the same pattern, another might be concerned about access for the poor, still another may be nervous about disagreeing with the medical society. Be sensitive to their distinctive concerns, and bring in individuals to talk with them who can answer those concerns. Your lobbyist can help you to determine the best way to approach various people. Pay special attention to those individuals who are identified as leaders in the legislature.

You may also need to rethink your strategy at any time. The psychologists from Louisiana have a number of stories of making decisions on the fly in response to a changing legislative picture, rushing from one house of the legislature to the other on a moment's notice or having to quickly undo damage done by the opponents to the bill.

LOOSE LIPS SINK SHIPS

Be careful about how much you reveal of your strategy. Assume that e-mail lists are open to spies from the opposition. If there is any possible benefit to keeping information private, then do so.

WIN THE WAR, SECURE THE PEACE

Imagine you reach a point at which the legislature has passed the bill and the governor has signed it. You may think at this point the time has come to lay down your weapons and bask in the thanks of a grateful nation. Such is not the case. The fact that no psychologist in Guam has ever written a prescription, even though prescriptive authority was achieved 10 years ago, illustrates the importance of the legislative process. In New Mexico, implementation was complicated by a clause in the law that assigns development of the regulations to a joint committee of the psychology and medical licensing boards. Even if the law assigns responsibility for the regulations to the psychology board, the results can be undesirable if the members of the licensing board are skeptical of prescriptive authority. It is wise to try to get supporters of RxP assigned to the licensing board before the legislation is passed in preparation for the development of the regulatory process.

Various other issues are likely to come up once prescriptive authority is achieved. To offer just a couple of examples: Insurance companies may be hesitant to reimburse, problems with the use of certain procedure codes not normally associated with psychologists can emerge, hospitals may refuse to allow psychologists to practice at a level consistent with their new authority, and psychologists must become part of whatever system the state uses to confirm eligibility for registration with the Drug Enforcement Agency. Problems with the law or regulations may become quickly evident and require additional changes. A good deal of work lies ahead. Do not put down that gun too quickly.

KEEP YOUR HEAD WHEN EVERYONE
ABOUT YOU IS LOSING THEIRS

Above all else, it is important to approach the process with humor and good sense. If you expect legislators to simply fall over at the rightness of giving psychologists prescriptive authority, you will be sorely disappointed. You must be ready to accept the losses and move on as well as to celebrate the victories. It will take a good deal of stamina to make it through the process, but the ultimate goal is worth it.

A CALL TO ACTION

This is a time of great foment among the health care and mental health care professions. Nurses are pursuing expansion of the scope of practice for nurse practitioners and nurse anesthetists in many states. The profession has a long-term commitment to advocating for the doctorate in nursing practice to become the basis for independent primary care practice. Optometrists who achieved prescriptive authority not too long ago are now asking for the authority to perform certain ocular surgeries. Master's level counselors are seeking to expand their capacity to practice independently in many states. Psychologists who are seeking prescriptive authority are not alone in their interest in using the legislative process to enhance the quality of service they can provide to their patients.

As I hope you can now appreciate, seeing an RxP bill through from beginning to end can be a long, frustrating, and arduous process. It can also be a very personally and professionally rewarding one. The prescriptive authority movement in psychology needs more generals. It needs leaders who are not afraid to stand up for the profession and will not succumb to the pressures from its well-organized and well-funded opposition. The movement also needs more captains, lieutenants, sergeants, and privates. Without hardworking soldiers in the trenches, a general's vision is just that: a vision.

That being said, getting involved in the prescriptive authority movement is not a difficult task. Most state psychological associations have active RxP committees that would appreciate your commitment of time and—yes—money. Divisions of the APA such as Division 55 (American Society for the Advancement of Pharmacotherapy); Division 18 (Psychologists in Public Service); and Division 19 (Society for Military Psychology) have active RxP committees, subcommittees, and educational and training opportunities. There are many who believe that RxP is important both for the opportunities it will create for our profession and for enhancing our ability to lobby for a more rational health care system. If you share these beliefs, it is time to join the fight.

13

THE FUTURE OF PRESCRIBING PSYCHOLOGY

BRET A. MOORE

This volume is a testament to decades of dedication, hard work, and success within a relatively small but highly influential group of professional psychologists. As we approach the 25th anniversary of Sen. Daniel K. Inouye's recommendation to the Hawaii Psychological Association that a paradigm shift occur in the profession, we are reminded of just how far the movement has come. Today, we reap the benefits of hard work and leadership in New Mexico, Louisiana, the Armed Forces, the U.S. Public Health Service, and the Indian Health Service (IHS). It is more important to note that the public reaps the benefits of a higher level of behavioral health care, particularly for those who are traditionally underserved (e.g., Native Americans), in need of targeted and immediate care (e.g., veterans and active duty military), and difficult to reach (e.g., rural communities). As one of the fathers of the prescriptive authority movement, Patrick DeLeon (2003), so aptly pointed out, "the prescriptive authority agenda is fundamentally a social policy agenda, that is, ensuring that all Americans have access to the highest possible quality of care" (p. xiii). This view remains particularly relevant, considering the current state of the economy and our military commitments.

Despite the successes in the prescriptive authority movement within professional psychology, there are areas that we need to continue to address. In this chapter, I highlight three such areas. First, I discuss issues related to professional practice. Second, I discuss issues related to the training and credentialing of prescribing–medical psychologists. Last, I highlight the importance of prescribing–medical psychologists taking more active and prominent roles in drug research.

PRACTICE ISSUES

Moving Into Traditional Medical Roles

Prescribing–medical psychologists who are moving into clinical and administrative positions traditionally held by medical professionals is a logical extension of psychologists' gaining of prescriptive authority. Even with a doctoral degree followed by a postdoctoral master's degree or certificate in clinical psychopharmacology, prescribing–medical psychologists come from a discipline that is often considered ancillary within the medical system. Like other disciplines that are considered ancillary (e.g., optometrists, podiatrists, clinical pharmacists), prescribing psychologists will face a struggle in their efforts to play a central role in health care decision making.

The fastest route prescribing–medical psychologists can take to break away from this professionally limiting categorization is to move into roles typically held by physicians, particularly psychiatrists. For example, the highest behavioral health positions in the U.S. Army tend to be held by psychiatrists, with the position of Clinical Psychology Consultant to the U.S. Army Surgeon General being the exception. Prescribing–medical psychologists, whether active duty or federal civilian employees, are in a unique position to challenge the long-held and misguided belief that physicians are the "quintessential" health care provider, particularly when it comes to behavioral health. Even psychologists without prescriptive authority are in as good or even better position to fill behavioral health leadership roles in the military, considering the extensive training we possess in understanding the psychological principles that underlie behavioral and psychological disturbances as well as the application of evidence-based methods to alleviate those problems.

Another instance in which prescribing–medical psychologists are in a good position to move into jobs typically held by traditional medical professionals in a federal agency may be found within the IHS. IHS is a division of the U.S. Department of Health and Human Services and is responsible for providing health and public services to American Indians and Alaskan Natives. Psychologists are employed as part of the U.S. Public Health Service and as federal civilian employees, and they occupy a variety of clinical and administrative positions. However, many of the high-level positions related to behavioral health are held by other medical professionals rather than psychologists. To the credit of IHS, this pattern is starting to change. At the time of this writing, the Phoenix, AZ, area behavioral health consultant is a Public Health Service psychologist, and the Billings, MT, area is actively seeking a psychologist to fill the position of its behavioral health consultant. In addition, the Billings area office is recruiting psychologists who are supportive of prescriptive authority for psychologists.

As important as the positions that psychologists hold in IHS, or any non-military federal position for that matter, is achieving status appropriate to our training and gaining parity with physicians with regard to salary. Much of the rationale for providing psychiatrists with higher salaries on the government service pay scale reflects psychiatrists' ability to generate more revenue than psychologists through medication services. Once more prescribing–medical psychologists enter federal agencies such as the IHS and provide medication management services, this argument starts to become less relevant. However, there are other factors that must be addressed before billing parity can be achieved, such as addressing private insurance and Medicaid–Medicare reimbursement rates for prescribing–medical psychologists.

How does this shift happen? First, prescribing–medical psychologists must dispense with the "ancillary provider mentality." For too long, psychologists have been relegated to a status within health care that does not recognize their skills and abilities. As a result of lower insurance reimbursement rates and exclusion from higher level clinical and administrative positions, we have learned to limit our objectives. It has to stop. Second, prescribing–medical psychologists must apply for administrative positions when they become available. Even if the position announcement states that a medical degree is required, apply anyway. The worst that can happen is that the application is rejected, but you never know the outcome. If no physicians apply and the position is generally a difficult one to fill, then someone with some pull and know-how may be able to get the position's requirements changed. Finally, get to know the people in your human resources department. In many organizations, they possess the knowledge about how to create new position descriptions and can assist with developing positions specific for prescribing–medical psychologists.

Expanding the Formulary

The next logical step in the evolution of psychological medicine is allowing prescribing–medical psychologists trained in neuropsychology and clinical health psychology as well as psychopharmacology to prescribe medications for the disorders typical to their practice. For example, a neuropsychologist should be allowed to prescribe acetylcholinesterase inhibitors for the treatment of Alzheimer's disease and dopamine-receptor agonists for the treatment of Parkinson's disease; a clinical health psychologist should be able to prescribe medications for the treatment of nicotine dependence, obesity, and diabetes.

Without question, this is a controversial topic, even among prescribing–medical psychologists. This controversy is understandable, considering that the prescriptive authority movement in general has many more battles ahead. However, as has been noted by several prominent proponents of the movement, the debate about whether appropriately trained psychologists can and should be able to prescribe is over. It is time to look toward the future.

Expanding the formulary for psychologists is not a new topic. As early as 1981, the American Psychological Association Board of Professional Affairs (1981) decided that any physical intervention relevant to the care of the patients they see should ultimately fall within the scope of practice of psychology so long as psychologists received the appropriate training and it was in the best interests of the patient. Earles, James, and Folen (2006) made a compelling argument for why clinical health psychologists with relevant training in psychopharmacology should be allowed to manage the more common medical disorders with strong behavioral and psychological components that are regularly seen in primary care clinics. Considering the high rates of death linked to obesity, tobacco use, and diabetes-related cardiovascular and kidney disease, the positive impact on society could be tremendous if the scope of prescriptive practice for appropriately trained psychologists were extended.

TRAINING

Internship and Postdoctoral Training

The standard training for prescribing–medical psychologists is at the postdoctoral and postlicensure level in the form of a master's degree or certificate. At a minimum, this ensures that psychologists have met the basic requirements for their profession and have some level of experience in providing behavioral and psychological interventions for the treatment of psychiatric disorders. In addition, many doctoral programs in psychology are providing exposure, although minimal, to students in clinical psychopharmacology. Should we be doing more?

In short, the answer is yes. As more states pass laws allowing psychologists to prescribe, the need for training is going to skyrocket. Students will start gravitating toward doctoral programs that include strong training in psychopharmacology. It is my hope that the supply will meet the demand.

In addition to academic coursework at the doctoral level, training at the internship level will need to occur as well. Rotations in clinical psychopharmacology will need to be created. To take it a step further, it is not unreasonable to incorporate psychopharmacology into existing clinical rotations, such as child and family psychology, behavioral medicine–health psychology, forensics, and substance abuse. Completing a 3-month rotation, shadowing a psychiatrist, prescribing–medical psychologist, or other relevant health care provider will provide an introductory level of exposure to the student and facilitate a smooth transition into postdoctoral training.

As noted earlier, postdoctoral training in clinical psychopharmacology occurs at the master's degree or certificate level. Establishing formal 2-year postdoctoral fellowships in clinical psychopharmacology can help augment this training. Collaborations between clinical sites and schools can create an optimal training environment in that students will be able to complete all three levels of psychopharmacology training at the same site during the fellowship period. Such opportunities are likely to emerge as states authorize prescriptive authority for psychologists.

One last issue in training has to do with the development of subspecialty tracks within psychopharmacology. Creating subspecialty tracks in training programs for psychologists with previous training in neuropsychology, clinical health psychology, child psychology, and geriatric psychology will help to advance the goal of moving prescribing–medical psychologists into primary care and long-term residential and neurorehabilitation settings.

Specialty Certification

Specialty certification provides peer and public recognition of competence and expertise in a specialty area of practice. It assures the public that the professional possesses skills and abilities beyond the basic level that are required for practice.

In psychology, the premier organization for certification in psychology is the American Board of Professional Psychology (ABPP). The ABPP currently provides certification in 13 separate areas of professional psychology: child and adolescent, clinical, clinical health, clinical neuropsychology, cognitive and behavioral, counseling, couple and family, forensic, group, organizational and business, psychoanalysis, rehabilitation, and school.

A logical step in solidifying the practice of clinical psychopharmacology as a mainstream practice in the field is to develop a certification board, and the ABPP is a logical organization to oversee that certification. Similar to the board certification in clinical psychology, requiring a credentials review to ensure that the candidate has met the academic and training requirements for practice in this area and completion of a written practice sample and oral examination would indicate skill and knowledge beyond the basic level. As with the other certifications, the general public would be assured that the psychologist has been judged by his or her peers as possessing an above-average level of competency. Some effort has been applied to developing a proposal for an ABPP related to psychologists' involvement in pharmacotherapy, but the initiative is still in a preliminary stage.

GETTING INVOLVED WITH DRUG RESEARCH

The foundation of psychology, and all sciences for that matter, is research. Without knowledge gleaned from research, psychologists would have little in the way of evidence-based treatments for psychiatric disorders. Consequently, one could argue that behavioral and psychological interventions would not be as effective as they are today.

Because psychology has such a rich history in the scientific method, it only makes sense that psychologists would take more of a lead in drug research. Much of the research done with psychotropic medications today involves psychiatrists in academic settings. This has more to do with the fact that psychologists have generally had limited access to opportunities in drug research than with level of preparedness to conduct research.

As more psychologists gain prescriptive authority, we should see a shift in this pattern. However, it is important for psychologists, whether trained in clinical psychopharmacology or not, to actively seek out research grants that involve clinical trials of new and existing psychotropics, volunteer their expertise for drug trials, and submit critiques to journals on research articles that report incorrect and misleading conclusions in regard to outcome. Basically, it is just a matter of expanding our knowledge, skills, and time in an area where we are already actively involved.

A FEW FINAL THOUGHTS

Prescribing psychology has come a long way. So many strides have been made over the past 3 decades, with tremendous gains manifesting just in the last several years. However, we still have a way to go.

Prescriptive authority has changed and will continue to change the face of professional psychology. The prescriptive authority movement is much larger than a few psychologists looking to write prescriptions. It is a shift in how we as professionals look at the practice of psychology as well as a shift in how the public views the profession.

In the near future, roles for many psychologists will change because of the prescriptive authority movement. Opportunities will open up that were once unavailable and the controversy over whether or not psychologists can or should prescribe will fade. The future appears bright.

REFERENCES

American Psychological Association Board of Professional Affairs. (1981). *Task force report: Psychologists' use of physical interventions.* Washington, DC: American Psychological Association.

DeLeon, P. H. (2003). Reflections on prescriptive authority and the evolution of psychology in the 21st century. In M. T. Sammons, R. F. Levant, & R. U. Paige (Eds.), *Prescriptive authority for psychologists: A history and guide* (pp. xi–xxiv). Washington, DC: American Psychological Association.

Earles, J. E., James, L. C., & Folen, R. A. (2006). Prescribing non-psychopharmaco-logical agents: A new potential role for psychologists in primary care settings and specialty clinics. *Journal of Clinical Psychology, 62,* 1213–1220. doi:10.1002/jclp.20304

INDEX

Aberdeen Area Indian Health Service, 212–214

Abilify, 143–145

Abnormal Involuntary Movement Scale (AIMS), 76

ABPP (American Board of Professional Psychology), 237–238

Absolute efficacy, 141

Absolute rate of improvement, 148

Academic problems, 196

Academy of Medical Psychology, 176

Accreditation, of institutions, 35, 37, 40, 42–43

Acetylcholinesterase inhibitors, 236

ACNP. *See* American College of Neuropsychopharmacology

Activating effect (of antidepressants), 136

Active-working phase (psychobiosocial model of care), 108, 115–118
    for individuals with severe mental illness, 124–125
    and use of antidepressants, 127

Acute care, in primary care psychology, 174, 175

Addictive problems, 168

ADHD. *See* Attention-deficit/ hyperactivity disorder

Adherence, 81. *See also* Compliance

Administration of medications, to school-aged patients, 202–203

Administrative positions, 235

Adolescents, 100, 106. *See also* School-aged patients

Advocates, patients as, 97

Age, of patients, 97

AIMS (Abnormal Involuntary Movement Scale), 76

Alaskan Natives (Native Alaskans), 209–214, 234

Albee, George, 86

Alliances, for RxP bills, 228

Alliant International University, 212

Allopathy, xiii

Ally, Glenn, 98–99

α level (α probability), 135, 136

Alzheimer's disease, 236

AMA (American Medical Association), 50

American Academy of Child and Adolescent Psychiatry, 198, 202

American Academy of Pediatrics, 200, 202

American Board of Professional Psychology (ABPP), 237–238

American College of Neuropsychopharmacology (ACNP), 20, 50, 52, 59–61

American Heart Association, 200

American Indians, 11, 209–214, 233–234

American Medical Association (AMA), 50

American Psychiatric Association, 15, 92

American Psychological Association (APA)
    on collaboration, 90
    curricula recommendations of, 30–42, 61
    model curriculum for prescriptive authority (2008), 18
    on pharmaceutical representatives, 3, 166
    and Psychology Demonstration Project, 50
    and reimbursement from Medicare/Medicaid, 176, 177
    and RxP bills, 224–226, 228
    training program evaluations by, 42–45

American Psychological Association Insurance Trust (APAIT), 21, 22, 74–75

American Society for the Advancement of Pharmacotherapy. *See* APA Division 55

American Society for the Advancement of Pharmacotherapy (APA Division 55), 91, 212, 225, 229, 232

Ancillary provider mentality, 235

Anderson, B. R., 178
Anorexia, 114
Answering services, 167
Antidepressants
    and Abilify, 143–145
    activating effect of, 136
    black box warnings for, 100,
        125–128
    and patient empowerment, 162
    prevalence of, 106
    tricyclic, 200
Antipsychotics, 115, 123, 146, 199, 200
Anxiety, 105, 117, 119–120, 161–162
APA. *See* American Psychological
    Association
APA Ad Hoc Task Force on Psycho-
    pharmacology, 31–33
APA Board of Educational Affairs, 61
APA Board of Professional Affairs, 236
APA College of Professional
    Psychology, 215
APA Commission on Specialties and
    Proficiencies, 32
APA Committee for the Advancement
    of Professional Practice
    (CAPP), 32
APA Committee for the Advancement
    of Professional Psychology,
    175, 225
APA Continuing Education
    Committee, 37
APA Council of Representatives, 34,
    43, 93
APA Division 18 (Psychologists in
    Public Service), 92, 212, 232
APA Division 19 (Society for Military
    Psychology), 232
APA Division 55 (American Society for
    the Advancement of Pharmaco-
    therapy), 91, 212, 225,
    229, 232
APA Ethics Code, 42, 93
APAIT. *See* American Psychological
    Association Insurance Trust
APA Practice Directorate, 61
APA Task Force on the Assessment
    of Competence in Professional
    Psychology, 42
Appetite suppressants, 114, 200
Appointment structures, 179

Aripiprazole, 143–145
Assessments. *See also* Evaluation(s)
    in practice guidelines, 95
    in psychobiosocial model of care, 110
    of school-aged patients, 195–197, 199
Atomoxetine, 200
Attention-deficit/hyperactivity disorder
    (ADHD), 105–106, 191, 193,
    196–197
Attitude, 232
Authorization, from insurance
    companies, 163–164
Autonomy, of patients, 117, 124–125

Barclay, A. G., 30, 52
BASC. *See* Behavior Assessment
    System for Children
BASC-Monitor, 199
Battle fatigue, 51, 53–54
BCRS (Bureau of Clinician Recruitment
    and Service), 208
Behavioral assessments, 196–197, 199
Behavioral techniques, 120
Behavior Assessment System for
    Children (BASC), 196, 199
Benzodiazepines, 83
Benztropine, 201
Berman, R. M., 143–144
Bias, in drug research, 133–134, 148
Biopsychosocial approach (biopsycho-
    social model of care). *See also*
    Psychobiosocial model of care
    in practice guidelines, 98
    in primary care, 178
    in private practice, 167, 170
    in training, 45
Bipolar disorder, 143, 197
Black box warnings
    and principle of least effect, 100
    and psychobiosocial model of care,
        125–128
    and school-aged patients, 198
Blount, A., 178
Blue Ribbon Panel
    and Psychology Demonstration
        Project, 50–54
    training recommendations of,
        32–33
Borderline personality disorder, 82
Brown, A. B., 51

Bryan, C., 126
Buelow, G. D., 91
Bureau of Clinician Recruitment and Service (BCRS), 208
Business issues, in prescriptive practice, 75–76

California, 11, 154
CAPP (APA Committee for the Advancement of Professional Practice), 32
Cardiovascular monitoring, 200
Care. *See also* Primary care; Psychobiosocial model of care
    acute, 174, 175
    coordinated and colocated, 178
    integrated, 174–175, 178
    quality of, 13–15, 97–98
Caregivers, of school-aged patients, 191–194, 196, 200–201
CBCL. *See* Child Behavior Checklist
CBT. *See* Cognitive behavioral therapy
CE. *See* Continuing education
Centers for Medicare & Medicaid Services, 176
Certification, 32, 237–238
Chafetz, M. D., 91
Charts, patient, 76, 79–80
CHCs (community health centers), 209
"Chemical imbalance," 113
Child Behavior Checklist (CBCL), 196, 199
Children. *See also* School-aged patients
    with anxiety disorders and ADHD, 105–106
    black box warnings for, 100, 126
    prevalence of mental health disorders in, 10
CIs (confidence intervals), 141–142
Citizens' Commission on Graduate Medical Education, 174
Civil Service, 210
Claymore-Lahammer, Vickie, 212
Clinical experience, 38, 40, 41, 45, 52, 237
Clinical health psychology, 235, 236
Clinical issues, in prescriptive practice, 75–76
Clinical medicine, 97–98

Clinical practicum, 35–37
Clinical privileges, xiii
Clinical psychopharmacology, 237
Clonazepam, 161, 162
CMHCs (community mental health centers), 209
Coalitions, for RxP bills, 225–226
Cochrane Reviews, 134
Codes, procedure, 166, 176
Cognitive behavioral therapy (CBT), 105, 106
Cognitive bias, 134
Cognitive dissonance, xv, 100
Cohen, J., 141
Collaboration
    consultation-liaison model of, 31, 182, 183
    in Indian Health Service, 213
    with parents, 192–193
    with patients, 99, 113, 118
    with primary care physicians, 115, 164–165, 195
    with teenagers, 201–202
    in training, 31, 237
Colocated care, 178
Commissioned Corps, 207, 210, 214–218
Committees, in state legislatures, 226
Community health centers (CHCs), 209
Community mental health centers (CMHCs), 209
Community-outpatient practice, 184–186
Competency model of evaluation, 41–42
Compliance
    and anxiety, 117
    with non-physician prescribers, 16
    in prescriptive practice, 81–82
    in private practice, 167
    of school-aged patients, 193, 200–201
Concurrence requirements, 164–165
Confidence intervals (CIs), 141–142
Congress. *See* U.S. Congress
CONsolidated Standards Of Reporting Trials (CONSORT), 145–146
Consultation
    practice guidelines on, 95–96
    in primary care, 178–182
    in psychobiosocial model of care, 115

Consultation-liaison model
(of collaboration), 31, 182, 183
Consultation reports, 180–181
Contact hours, in training curricula, 33,
35–36
Continuing education (CE), 32, 37, 40,
166
Continuous performance tests (CPTs),
196–197
Control, locus of, 117–118, 121
Controlled Substance Registration
Certificate (DEA number), 73,
74, 166
Controlled substances, 76, 82–84,
193–194
Cooper, C., 81
Coordinated care, 178
Cordero, L., 126
Correlation coefficient, 138
Corso, K., 126
Costs
in prescriptive practice, 15,
85–86
in private practice, 166
of Psychology Demonstration
Project, 62
of RxP bills, 227–228
of training, 19, 20, 30
Counselors, 4, 232
Countertransference, 161–162
CPTs (continuous performance tests),
196–197
Credentialing, 64
Curriculum(-a)
evaluating, 44–45
Curriculum(-a)
for PDP, 50–58
recommendations for, 30–42

DEA. See Drug Enforcement Agency
DEA number. See Controlled Substance
Registration Certificate
deGruy, F., III, 177
DeLeon, P. H., 211, 233
Demand for mental health services, xiv,
5, 10
Department of Defense (DoD), 21,
208–209, 214–216. See also
Psychopharmacology Demonstra-
tion Project (PDP)

Department of Health and Human
Services (DHHS), 207, 208,
218, 234
Department of Homeland Security,
216–217
Department of Transportation, 217
Deployed settings, 64–65
Depression, 63, 106, 144–145,
162, 197
Designation Criteria for Education and
Training Programs in Preparation
for Prescriptive Authority (2009),
42–45
Developmental information, in medical
history, 194
Dextroamphetamine, 200, 202
DHHS. See Department of Health and
Human Services
Diagnoses, 14, 162
Diagnosis (diagnostic) phase
(psychobiosocial model of care),
108–111
for individuals with severe mental
illness, 123–124
and use of antidepressants, 126
Diagnostic and Statistical Manual of
Mental Disorders, 110
Didactic instruction (didactic training),
41, 45, 52, 57, 62
DIHS (Division of Immigration Health
Services), 216–217
Disaster mental health response teams
(MHTs), 211
Discontinuation of medication, 194
Diversion of medication, 193–194
Diversity factors, 32, 42
Division of Immigration Health Services
(DIHS), 216–217
Divorced parents, 193
Doctor–patient relationship, 97
Documentation (record keeping),
75–76, 79–80, 168
DoD. See Department of Defense
DoD-PHS Partners in Mental Health,
215, 216
Donaldson, M. S., 174
Dopamine-receptor agonists, 236
Dorken, Herbert, 154
Dosage, changing, 81
Draft bills, for RxP, 226

Drug companies. *See* Pharmaceutical companies
Drug Enforcement Agency (DEA), 73, 176, 231
Drug interactions, 78, 114–115, 118, 168
Drug (pharmaceutical) representatives, 76, 100, 165–166
Drug research, 133–149
  applications of, 143–145
  bias in, 133–134
  confidence intervals for, 141–142
  effect size statistics for, 137–141
  and patient withdrawal, 142–143
  and prescribing–medical psychologists, 238
  questions for interpreting, 145–148
  for school-aged patients, 197
  significance testing for, 135–137
Drug-seeking patients, 82–84
Duke, Tim, 20

Earles, J. E., 236
Economically disadvantaged patients, 12
Education. *See also* Training
  continuing, 32, 37, 40, 166
  practice guidelines on, 94
Effectiveness, 133n.1
Effect size, 137–141, 147
Efficacy
  effectiveness vs., 133n.1
  of medications for school-aged patients, 198–200
  relative vs. absolute, 140–141
Electrocardiograms (EKGs), 200
Emergency clinical responders, 212
Emotional disorders, 196
Emotional disturbance, 21–22
Empowerment, of patients, 162
Engagement, in training programs, 45
Escitalopram, 162
"Ethical Principles of Psychologists and Code of Conduct" (American Psychological Association), 42, 93
Ethics, 89–101
  of pharmaceutical marketing, 99–101
  practice guidelines on, 91–96
  in professional relationships, 101

  in psychological model of prescribing, 98–99
  and psychologists' knowledge of medications, 93, 96–98
  and three levels of involvement, 90
Evaluation(s)
  competency model of, 41–42. *See also* Assessments
  intake, 75
  school-based, 190–191
  of side effects, 118, 119
Expectations, of patients, 77–78
Expertise, 84
Extrapyramidal symptoms, 76

FDA. *See* Food and Drug Administration
Federal Bureau of Prisons, 217
"File drawer problems," 148
Final Report of the Board of Educational Affairs (BEA) Working Group to Develop a Level 1 Curriculum for Psychopharmacology Education and Training (American Psychological Association), 33
Final Report of the Board of Educational Affairs (BEA) Working Group to Develop Curriculum for Level 2 Training in Psychopharmacology (American Psychological Association), 33
Fluoxetine, 126, 193
Folen, R. A., 236
Food and Drug Administration (FDA), 125, 126, 133, 147, 148, 197, 198
Formularies, 163, 235–236
Fox, R. E., 30, 32
Freud, Sigmund, 128–129
"Frontier" areas, 208
Full service providers, 169
Fundraising, for RxP bills, 227–228

Gaissmaier, W., 141
GAO. *See* General Accounting Office
Garcia, Joxel, 214
General Accounting Office (GAO), 19, 59–61
Generalization phase (psychobiosocial model of care), 108, 118–121

Generalization phase, *continued*
    for individuals with severe mental
        illness, 125
    and use of antidepressants, 127
Generals (for RxP bills), 225
Geraghty, E. M., 63
Gift giving, by pharmaceutical
        companies, 99–100
Gigerenzer, G., 141
Goals, of consultants vs. specialists,
        179
Goldberg, T. E., 146
Goodman, "Maury," 153
Governors, support of RxP bills from,
        228
Grants, for RxP bills, 225, 228
Grill, D. J., 52
Guam, 231
Guidelines Regarding Psychologists'
    Involvement in Pharmacological
    Issues (APA Council of
        Representatives), 93–96

Hatfield, D. R., 81
Haug, J. D., 100
Hawaii, 10–11
Hawaii Psychological Association, 233
Health and Behavior Assessment and
        Intervention procedure codes,
        176
Health care
    and Indian Health Service, 211
    psychologists as providers of, 173, 186
    psychology's contributions to, 175
    for veterans, 153
Health insurance, 153–154
Health literacy, of patients, 97
Health maintenance organizations
        (HMOs), 63
Health professional shortage areas
        (HPSAs), 209
Health Resources and Services Admin-
        istration (HRSA), 207–209
Hearings, legislative, 229–230
Heiser, Karl, 153
HMOs (health maintenance
        organizations), 63
Hollon, S. D., 106
Hopewell, Alan, 20
Hospitalist system, 185

Hospitals
    implementation of RxP bills, 231
    prescribing in, 78, 177
    primary care, 182–184
    privileges for psychologists, 154
HPSAs (health professional shortage
        areas), 209
HRSA (Health Resources and Services
        Administration), 207–209

ICD 9 (International Classification of
        Diseases), 110
Identity, 22, 71–72
IHS. *See* Indian Health Service
IHS Behavioral Health Program, 210
Immigration and Customs
        Enforcement, 216
Implementation (of RxP bills), 231
Improvement, absolute rate of, 148
Income, 166
Indian Health Service (IHS)
    prescribing in, 11, 52, 71, 234–235
    and Public Health Service, 209–214
Information products, of consultants vs.
        specialists, 180
Informed consent, 79, 91, 113–114,
        167, 183
Inouye, Daniel K., 50, 233
Inpatient mental health services,
        54–55, 80
Institutions, accreditation of, 35, 37,
        40, 42–43
Insurance
    health, 153–154, 163–164, 170, 231
    liability, 21, 22, 74–75
Intake evaluations, 75
Integrated care, 174–175, 178
Integrated mental health services,
        13–15
Integrated Visual–Auditory Plus, 196
Interactions, drug, 78, 114–115, 118,
        168
International Classification of Diseases
        (ICD 9), 110
Internships, 34–35, 236–237
Interpersonal therapy, 106
Interpretation of Dreams (Sigmund
        Freud), 128–129
Interventions, 4, 95–96, 179
Interviews, for medical histories, 195

Involvement, three levels of, 90
Irving and Dorothy Rom Family
    Foundation, 212

James, L. C., 236
JCAH (Joint Commission for the
    Accreditation of Hospitals),
    154
Jennings, Floyd, 52, 210, 211
Joint Commission for the Accreditation
    of Hospitals (JCAH), 154
"Junior psychiatrists," 5

Kessler, R. C., 10
Knowledge, about medications, 93,
    96–98
Krupnick, J. L., 112
Kurz-Milcke, E., 141

Lakota Sicangu tribe, 211
LAMP. See Louisiana Academy of
    Medical Psychologists
Laskow, G. B., 52
Lasser, K. E., 147
Last observation carried forward
    (LOCF) analysis, 142–143
Learning problems, 191, 196
Legislation. See Prescriptive authority
    legislation for psychologists
    (RxP)
Legislative hearings, on RxP bills,
    229–230
Legislative support, for RxP bills,
    229–231
Leigh, H., 183
Level 1 training, 31, 33, 90
Level 2 training, 31, 33, 90
Level 3 training, 31, 90
LeVine, Elaine, 154, 161
Lexapro, 162
Liability insurance, 21, 22, 74–75
Licensed counselors, 4
Licensing
    boards for, 72, 228
    costs of, 166
    in Indian Health Service, 213
    and postdoctoral training, 34–35
    and private practice, 153
    in Public Health Service, 208–209
Lipsey, M. W., 146

Lobbyists, 226–228, 230–231
LOCF analysis. See Last observation
    carried forward analysis
Locus of control, 117–118, 121
Lohr, K. N., 174
Louisiana
    medical psychologists in, 72–73,
        175–176
    prescriptive authority in, 11–13,
        154
    private practice in, 154–170
    RxP initiatives in, 225, 231
    safety of prescribing psychologists in,
        21
Louisiana Academy of Medical
    Psychologists (LAMP), 73, 74
Louisiana Association of Medical
    Psychologists, 225
Louisiana Board of Psychologist
    Examiners, 154
Louisiana Controlled and Dangerous
    Substance License, 73n.1

MADRS (Montgomery–Åsberg Depres-
    sion Rating Scale), 144–145
Maintenance sessions, 122, 123
Major depressive disorders (MDD), 126
Malpractice, 21, 22
Managed care companies, 163–164,
    166, 170
Marcus, S., 106
Marketing, by pharmaceutical
    companies, 99–101
Marquez, Mario, 154
McGrath, R. E., 16–18, 64–65, 91
MDD (major depressive disorders),
    126
Medicaid, 13, 74, 170, 176, 177, 235
Medical education model (of training),
    55–59
Medical Expenditures Panel Surveys,
    106
Medical histories, of school-aged
    patients, 194–195
Medical model, 110, 116–118, 164, 177
Medical psychologists. See also
        Prescribing–medical psychologists
    biopsychosocial model of care for,
        106–107
    as emergency clinical responders, 212

Medical psychologists, *continued*
  in hospital settings, 177
  in Louisiana, 72–73
  in Public Health Service. *See* Public
    Health Service (PHS)
  roles of, 178–186
  school-aged patients of. *See* School-
    aged patients
Medical psychology, 18, 175–178
Medical records, 75–76
Medical roles (for prescribing–medical
  psychologists), 234–235
Medical school argument, 15–19
Medicare, 170, 176, 177, 235
Medicare Improvements for Patients
  and Providers Act of 2008, 170
Medication
  administration and preparation of,
    202–203
  discontinuation of, 194
  historical use of, 105–107
  preparing patients for, 78–79
  psychologists' knowledge of, 93,
    96–98
  risk–benefit analysis of, 147
  for school-aged patients, 189–190,
    198–200
  as transference object, 116, 117
  as transitional object, 121, 122
  weaning from, 81
Medication management, 97, 163, 164,
  167, 170, 235
Medicine
  prescriptive authority in, xiii–xiv
  training for, 17, 18
Mental disorders, prevalence of, 10
Mental health services
  demand for, xiv, 5, 10
  inpatient, 54–55, 80
  integrated, 13–15
  outpatient, 54
Mental health specialists, 178–182
Mental illness, severe, 123–125, 163
Meta-analysis, 137–138
Metabolic syndrome, 115, 123
Methylphenidate, 200, 202
MHTs (disaster mental health response
  teams), 211
Midlevel practitioners, 73–74

Military patients, 63–65, 233. *See also*
  Department of Defense; Psycho-
  pharmacology Demonstration
  Project (PDP)
Military readiness, 19–20
Misdiagnosis, 18
Monitoring, 80–81, 199, 200
Montana Area Indian Health Service,
  213, 214
Montgomery–Åsberg Depression Rating
  Scale (MADRS), 144–145
Mood-stabilizing agents, 199, 200
Moore, B., 64–65
Mortality gap, 123
Murtha, John, 51
Muse, M., 16–18

National Alliance on Mental Illness,
  228
National disasters, 211
National Health Service Corps
  (NHSC), 208
Native Alaskans (Alaskan Natives),
  209–214, 234
Native Americans (American Indians),
  11, 209–214, 233–234
Neuropsychology, 235–236
New Jersey, 153–154
New Mexico
  Indian Health Service in, 210, 211
  prescribing psychologists in,
    11–13, 72
  prescriptive authority in, 154
  private practice in, 154–170
  RxP bills in, 231
  safety of prescribing psychologists
    in, 21
  training in, 18
New Mexico Board of Psychologist
  Examiners, 154
New Mexico Psychological Association,
  210–211
NHSC (National Health Service
  Corps), 208
NNT (number needed to treat),
  140–141
No effect (in drug research), 135
Null hypothesis, 135–137
Number needed to treat (NNT), 140–141
Nursing, 4, 17, 18, 52–53, 232

Observed cases (OC) analysis, 142–143
Obsessive–compulsive disorder, 82
OC analysis. *See* Observed cases
    analysis
Odds ratio (OR), 139–140
Off-hour telephone calls, 167
Office of the Undersecretary of Defense
    for Health Affairs, 58–59
Off-label prescribing, 197–198
Ogles, B. M., 81
Ohio Psychological Association, 154
Olfson, M., 106
One-group, pretest–posttest design,
    146
Operation Iraqi Freedom, 64
Optometrists, 232
OR (odds ratio), 139–140
Oral contraceptives, 141
Oral interviews, for medical
    histories, 195
Oral medications, 202–203
Outpatient mental health services, 54
Overdiagnosis, 18

Panic disorder, 117
Parents, 191–196, 200–201
Parkinson's disease, 236
Paroxetine, 114
PAs. *See* Physician assistants
Patient charts, 76, 79–80
Patient-Recorded Outcomes Measure-
    ment Information System
    (PROMIS), 81
Patients. *See also* Military patients;
    School-aged patients
    as advocates, 97
    autonomy of, 117, 124–125
    collaboration with, 99, 113, 118
    drug-seeking, 82–84
    empowerment of, 162
    expectations of, 77–78
    locus of control for, 117–118
    of other prescribers, 84–85
    personality characteristics of, 82
    preparing, for medication, 78–79
    "problem," 78
    selecting, 76–78
    with severe mental illness, 123–125
    teenagers as, 201–202
    underserved, 10–13

Patient-specific factors, 114
Patient withdrawal, in drug research,
    142–143
Paxil, 162
PCPs. *See* Primary care physicians
PDP. *See* Psychopharmacology
    Demonstration Project
Peck, B. M., 77
Pediatric psychology, 189. *See also*
    School-aged patients
PediSure, 200
PEP. *See* Psychopharmacology Examina-
    tion for Psychologists
Personal digital assistants, 80
Personality characteristics, of patients, 82
Pharmaceutical companies
    drug research from, 143, 145. *See also*
        Drug research
    marketing by, 99–101
    relationships with, 165–166
Pharmaceutical (drug) representatives,
    76, 100, 165–166
Pharmacotherapy, 3–4. *See also* Psycho-
    biosocial model of care
Phi coefficient, 138
PHS. *See* Public Health Service
Physician assistants (PAs), 52–53
Physicians, 16, 174, 228, 234. *See also*
    Primary care physicians (PCPs)
Placebos, 135–140, 146
Point-biserial correlation, 138
Polypharmacy, 91, 155, 197–198
Population effects, 137
Postdoctoral training
    APA recommendations for, 34–42
    for prescribing–medical psychol-
        ogists, 236–237
    *Recommended Postdoctoral Education
        and Training Program in Psycho-
        pharmacology for Prescriptive
        Authority* (2009), 38–42
    *Recommended Postdoctoral Training in
        Psychopharmacology for Prescrip-
        tion Privileges* (1996), 34–37
    in *Report of the Blue Ribbon Panel*, 33
Potency, 148
Power (in significance testing), 136–137
Practicum
    clinical, 35–37
    supervised, 30–31, 33, 35–37

Preferred Reporting Items for System-
        atic Reviews and Meta-Analyses
        (PRISMA), 146
Pregnancy, 202
Preparation(s)
    of medications for school-aged
        patients, 202–203
    of patients for medication, 78–79
    for prescriptive practice, 73–74
    for RxP bills, 226–227
Prescribing. *See* Psychological model of
        prescribing
Prescribing–medical psychologists,
        233–239. *See also* Private
        practice; Psychobiosocial model
        of care
    and drug research, 238
    formularies of, 235–236
    in medical roles, 234–235
    specialty certification of, 237–238
    training for, 236–237
    treatment of severe mental illness by,
        123–125
Prescribing proficiency, 32
Prescribing psychologists (term), 72.
        See also Prescribing–medical
        psychologists
Prescription pads, 74, 80
Prescriptive authority, 9–22
    current initiatives in, 61–63
    importance of, 4
    and medical school argument, 15–19
    psychologists' concerns about, 21–22
    and Psychology Demonstration
        Project, 19–20
    and psychology profession, xiii–xv
    and quality of care, 13–15
    risks of, 5–6
    safety of, 20–21
    and underserved populations, 10–13
Prescriptive authority legislation for
        psychologists (RxP), 223–232
    alliances for, 228
    attitude about, 232
    core coalitions for, 225–226
    fundraising for, 227–228
    generals for, 225
    implementation of, 231
    legislative hearings on, 229–230
    legislative support for, 229–231

    members' interest in, 224–225
    preparations for, 226–227
    revealing strategy for, 231
    time commitment for, 230
    and training, 227
Prescriptive practice, 71–86
    and area of expertise, 84
    clinical and business issues in, 75–76
    compliance in, 81–82
    deciding to begin, 85–86
    discussing side effects in, 79
    documenting prescriptions for, 79–80
    and drug-seeking patients, 82–84
    monitoring progress in, 80–81
    patient selection in, 76–78
    and patients of other prescribers,
        84–85
    preparing for, 73–74
    preparing patients for medication in,
        78–79
    and professional identity, 71–72
President's New Freedom Commission
        on Mental Health, 122
Primary care, 173–186
    in community-outpatient practice,
        184–186
    consultation in, 178–182
    defined, 174
    evolution of, 173–174
    in hospitals, 182–184
    interventions in, 4
    and medical psychology, 175–178
    and mental health care, 14
    and primary care psychology,
        174–175
    psychopharmacotherapy in, 10
Primary care associations, 228
Primary care behavioral health
        consultants, 178–182
Primary care physicians (PCPs)
    collaboration with, 115, 127,
        164–165, 185
    defined, 174
    and mental health consultants/
        specialists, 178–182
    and primary care psychology, 175
    referrals from, 162
    of school-aged patients, 195
    training of, 62–63
Primary care psychology, 174–175

Principle of least effect, 100
Principles of Medical Ethics (American
    Psychiatric Association), 92
Prior authorization, from insurance
    companies, 163–164
PRISMA (Preferred Reporting Items for
    Systematic Reviews and Meta-
    Analyses), 146
Private practice survey, 153–170
    anecdotes in, 161–169
    conclusions from, 169–170
    and evolution of private practice,
        153–154
    method of, 154–155
    results from, 155–161
"Problem patients," 78
Procedure codes, 166, 176
Professional relationships, 101
Proficiencies, 32, 40
PROMIS (Patient-Recorded Outcomes
    Measurement Information
    System), 81
Proposed Curriculum for Psychopharma-
    cology Training for Professional
    Psychologists (1992), 30
Pseudopsychiatric conditions, 97
Psychiatric services
    availability of, 11, 97
    demand for, xiv, 5, 10
Psychiatrists, 51–52, 62, 234
Psychiatry, 4, 21–22, 54
Psychobiosocial model of care, 105–129.
        See also Biopsychosocial approach
        (biopsychosocial model of care)
    active-working phase, 115–118
    and antidepressant black box
        warnings, 125–128
    diagnosis phase, 109–111
    generalization phase, 118–121
    and history of psychotropic
        treatment, 105–107
    for patients with severe mental
        illness, 123–125
    relationship-building phase, 111–115
    tenets of, 107–108
    termination phase, 121–123
Psychological model of prescribing
    diversity factors in, 32
    ethics in, 98–99
    medical model vs., xiv
    in practice guidelines, 91

Psychologists. *See also* Prescribing–
    medical psychologists
    as consumers of drug research, 134
    as full service providers, 169
    and knowledge of medications,
        93, 96–98
    opposition to prescriptive authority
        from, 50, 229
    as providers of health care, 173
Psychologists in Public Service (APA
    Division 18), 92, 212, 232
Psychology
    clinical health, 235, 236
    identity of, 22
    medical, 18, 175–178
    neuro-, 235–236
    pediatric, 189
    primary care, 174–175
    as profession, xiii–xv
    training for, 16–18
Psychopharmacology, 5, 237
Psychopharmacology Demonstration
    Project (PDP), 49–66
    controversy over, 49–50
    curriculum for, 50–58
    external scrutiny of, 58–61
    and prescribing for the military, 63–65
    prescribing psychologists in, 72
    and prescriptive authority, 19–20
    and prescriptive authority initiatives,
        61–63
    and Pubic Health Service, 214–216
Psychopharmacology Examination for
    Psychologists (PEP), 18, 71,
    215, 216
Psychopharmacotherapy, 10
Psychosocial factors, 21–22, 91
Psychosocial model of practice, 34, 42
Psychotherapy, pharmacotherapy and.
        See Psychobiosocial model of care
Publication bias, 148
Public Health Service (PHS), 207–218
    and Department of Defense,
        214–216
    and Department of Homeland
        Security, 216–217
    and Federal Bureau of Prisons, 217
    and Health Resources and Services
        Administration, 207–209
    and Indian Health Service, 209–214
p value, 135, 136

Quality of care, 13–15, 97–98
QUality Of Reporting Of Meta-analyses (QUOROM), 146
Quillin, James, 73
QUOROM (QUality Of Reporting Of Meta-analyses), 146

Randomized clinical trials (RCTs), 134–135. *See also* Drug research
Rao, N. R., 10
Ray, Oakley, 50
RCTs. *See* Randomized clinical trials
Ready Responders, 208–209
Recommended Postdoctoral Education and Training Program in Psychopharmacology for Prescriptive Authority (2009), 38–42
Recommended Postdoctoral Training in Psychopharmacology for Prescription Privileges (1996), 32–37
Record keeping. *See* Documentation
Recovery (in psychobiosocial model of therapy), 122
Recruitment, 213
Referrals
    and biopsychosocial model of prescribing, 98–99
    and income, 166
    from other psychologists, 84, 167
    from PCPs, 78, 162, 180, 185
    of school-aged patients, 190, 191
Reframing, 117–118
Regional accreditation, of institutions, 35, 37, 40, 42–43
Reimbursement
    and ancillary provider mentality, 235
    from Medicaid, 13
    for medication management, 163, 164
    in private practice, 166, 170
Relapse, 125
Relationship-building phase (psychobiosocial model of care), 108, 111–115
    for individuals with severe mental illness, 124
    and use of antidepressants, 127
Relationships
    doctor–patient, 97

with drug representatives, 100
    practice guidelines on, 96
    professional, 101
    therapeutic, 111–112, 127, 167–168
Relative efficacy, 140
Relative risk ratio (RR), 138, 139
Remeron, 162
Report of the Blue Ribbon Panel— Professional Education Task Force of the California Psychological Association and the California School of Professional Psychology, 32–33
Resiliency factors, 107, 108
Responsibility of prescribing, 161–162
Right to unprescribe, 155
Risk–benefit analysis, for medication, 147
Risperidone, 198
Rom-Rymer, Beth, 92
Rosebud Nation, 211
RR. *See* Relative risk ratio
Rudd, M., 126
Runyan, C. N., 178
Rural areas, 11, 208, 233
RxP. *See* Prescriptive authority legislation for psychologists

Safety, xv, 20–21, 198
Sammons, M. T., 51
Samples (from drug representatives), 76, 165–166
Sample size (for drug research), 146–147
Schizophrenia, 123, 143, 146
School-aged patients, 189–203. *See also* Children
    and black box warnings, 198
    compliance of, 200–201
    drug administration and preparation for, 202–203
    efficacy of medications for, 198–200
    medical histories of, 194–195
    off-label prescribing and polypharmacy for, 197–198
    parents of, 191–194
    primary care physicians of, 195
    psychotropic medication for, 189–190

school-based evaluations of, 190–191

standardized assessments of, 195–197

teenagers as, 201–202

School-based evaluations (of school-aged patients), 190–191

Schwartz, L. M., 141

Schwelitz, F. D., 30

Scientist–practitioner model, 34

Sedatives, 78, 114–115

Selective serotonin reuptake inhibitors (SSRIs), 80–81, 114, 119, 120, 193

Self-observation, 118–120

Sensorium, 136

Sertraline, 80, 105

Severe mental illness, 123–125, 163

Sexual dysfunction, 114

Shapiro, A. E. "Gene," 153

Sherman, Jeff, 216–217

Side effects

and compliance, 82

in drug research, 147

and informed consent, 79, 114

patients' evaluations of, 118, 119

practice guidelines on, 91

and psychobiosocial model of care, 105, 107–108

psychologists' knowledge of, 97

for school-aged patients, 197

Significance testing, for drug research, 135–137

Slate, Dennis, 216

Sleep problems, 194–195

Smyer, M. A., 5, 90, 92, 96n.1

Social stigma, 201–202

Social workers, 4

Society for Military Psychology (APA Division 19), 232

South Dakota, 211

Sponsors (of RxP bills), 227, 229

SSRIs. See Selective serotonin reuptake inhibitors

Standardized assessments, 195–197

Standardized mean difference, 138

Standards, in drug research, 145–146

STAndards for the Reporting of Diagnostic (STARD) accuracy studies, 146

State associations, RxP bills and, 224–225

State Controlled Substance Registration, 166

State legislatures, 226

State licensing boards, 72

Statins, 133

Stigma, social, 201–202

Stimulants, 198–200

Subspecialty tracks, 237

Substance abuse, 200

Suicidality (suicidal ideation), 100, 125–127

Supervised clinical experience, 38, 40, 41, 45

Supervised practicum, 30–31, 33, 35–37

Support, for RxP bills, 228–231

Surveys, 11–13. See also Private practice survey

Symptoms, extrapyramidal, 76

Taft-Hartley Act of 1947, 153

Teachers, 196

Teenagers, 201–202. See also Adolescents

Telephone calls, 80, 167

Telepsychiatry, 230

Tennessee, 11

Termination of therapy, 180

Termination phase (psychobiosocial model of care), 108, 121–123

for individuals with severe mental illness, 125

and use of antidepressants, 128

Test of Variables of Attention, 196

Therapeutic alliance (therapeutic relationship), 111–112, 127, 167–168

Time commitment, for RxP bills, 230

Training, 29–45. See also Postdoctoral training

in clinical medicine, 97–98

collaboration in, 31, 237

costs of, 19, 20, 30

designation criteria for training programs, 42–45

didactic, 41, 45, 52, 57, 62

history of, 30–33

and Indian Health Services, 212

Level 1, Level 2, and Level 3 training, 31, 33, 90

Training, *continued*
   medical education model of, 55–59
   at medical schools, 15–16
   in medication management, 97
   mission of, xiv–xv
   for nursing, medicine, and
      psychology, 16–18
   for prescriptive authority, 168–169
   of primary care physicians, 62–63
   and psychobiosocial model of care,
      107–108, 110, 113
   for Psychology Demonstration
      Project, 52, 54
   and RxP bills, 227
   triadic model of, 90
Transdermal patches, 202
Transference objects, 116, 117
Transitional objects, 121, 122
Treatment for Adolescents with
   Depression Study, 106
Triadic model of training, 90
Tribal governments, 210
Tricyclic antidepressants, 200
t statistic, 135
Two-condition case, 135
Type I error, 135
Type II error, 136

Underserved populations
   access for, 10–13
   private practice treatment for,
      162–163
   and Public Health Service, 208,
      209, 233
Uniformed Services University of the
   Health Sciences (USUHS)
   model, 53, 55

Unipolar depression, 197
Unprescribing, 155
Urban areas, 11, 209
U.S. Air Force, 64, 215
U.S. Air Force Medical Service, 178
U.S. Army, 55, 64, 216, 234
U.S. Coast Guard, 217
U.S. Congress, 50–51, 58, 60
U.S. Navy, 55, 64, 215
USUHS model. *See* Uniformed Services
   University of the Health Sciences
   model

Vacation coverage, 84–85
VandenBos, G. R., 90
Vaneslow, N. A., 174
Vector Research, 20
Veterans, 153, 215, 233
Vulnerability factors, 107, 108

Walkup, J. T., 105
Walter Reed Army Medical Center
   (WRAMC), 53, 55, 56
Weaning from medications, 81
Weight gain, 114, 199
Wiggins, Jack, 154
Williams, S., 90
Wilson, D. B., 146
Woloshin, S., 141
World War II, 153
WRAMC. *See* Walter Reed Army
   Medical Center

Yordy, K. D., 174

Zolpidem, 162

ABOUT THE EDITORS

Robert E. McGrath, PhD, is a professor of psychology at Fairleigh Dickinson University, where he currently directs both the doctoral program in clinical psychology and the master of science program in clinical psychopharmacology. He received his doctorate in clinical psychology in 1984 from Auburn University. He has since authored approximately 150 publications and presentations, primarily in the areas of assessment and measurement, statistical methodology, and professional issues in pharmacotherapy. Dr. McGrath has been a candidate for president of the American Psychological Association (APA), serves on the APA Division 12 (Society of Clinical Psychology) Committee on Science and Practice and is a former president of APA Division 55 (American Society for the Advancement of Pharmacotherapy). He is a three-time winner of the Martin Mayman Award presented by the Society for Personality Assessment for contributions to the literature on personality assessment.

Bret A. Moore, PsyD, ABPP, is a clinical psychologist with the Indian Health Service and a former active-duty Army psychologist. He received his doctorate in clinical psychology in 2004 from the Adler School of Professional Psychology, Chicago, Illinois, and his master's degree in clinical psycho-pharmacology in 2009 from Fairleigh Dickinson University. Dr. Moore is coeditor of *Living and Surviving in Harm's Way: A Psychological Treatment Handbook for Pre- and Post-Deployment of Military Personnel* and coauthor of *The Veterans and Active Duty Military Psychotherapy Treatment Planner*. He is an active member of American Psychological Association Division 55 (American Society for the Advancement of Pharmacotherapy), former membership chair for Division 18 (Psychologists in Public Service), and RxP chair for Division 19 (Society for Military Psychology).